Nursing in the UK

A Handbook for Nurses from Overseas and the EU

Nursing in the UK

A Handbook for Nurses from Overseas and the EU

Wendy Benbow and Gill Jordan

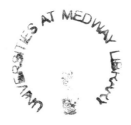

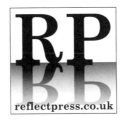

reflectpress.co.uk

© 2007, Wendy Benbow and Gill Jordan

The right of Wendy Benbow and Gill Jordan to be identified as authors of this work has been asserted by them in accordance with the Copyright, Designs and Patents Act 1988.

First published in 2007

ISBN: 978 1 906052 00 3

British Library Cataloguing in Publication Data
A catalogue record for this book is available from the British Library

The authors and publisher have made every attempt to ensure the content of this book is up-to-date and accurate. However, healthcare knowledge and information is changing all the time so the reader is advised to double-check any information in this text on drug usage, treatment procedures, the use of equipment, etc. to confirm that it complies with the latest safety recommendations, standards of practice and legislation. The publisher and authors accept no responsibility and assume no liability for any harm to persons or property resulting from the information and/or procedures in this textbook.

Production project management by Deer Park Productions

Typeset by Pantek Arts Ltd, Maidstone, Kent

Cover design by Oxmed

Printed and bound by Bell & Bain Ltd, Glasgow

Distributed by BEBC, Albion Close, Parkstone, Poole, Dorset BH12 3LL

www.reflectpress.co.uk

Published by Reflect Press Ltd
11 Attwyll Avenue
Exeter
Devon
EX2 5HN
UK
01392 204400

Contents

Introduction

The Nursing and Midwifery Council's (NMC) requirement for qualified nurses from overseas to undertake a period of study, and in some instances a period of supervised practice, became statutory in September 2005. Following completion of these elements, nurses are eligible to apply for inclusion on the NMC Register of Nurses. This handbook endeavours to act as a resource for the required 20 days of study element and is based on the NMC's (2005) prescribed content for the Overseas Nurses Programme (see Appendix, page 179). While it is only nurses from overseas who have to undertake an approved programme, it is envisaged that nurses from EU countries may also find the contents of this handbook helpful when nursing in the UK. Equally, nurses studying on a Return to Practice Programme should find it a good companion to their studies.

We were very conscious when writing this handbook that the readers will be registered nurses in their own countries and very probably have a wealth of nursing experience. Therefore the aim of this handbook is to help contextualise previous nursing experience in work as a registered practitioner within the 'culture' and environment of the UK health system. Some of the information will not be new and, where this happens, we would encourage you to view the topics as an update of the many important issues that relate to nursing practice. Owing to the range and nature of topics discussed, the chapters will interrelate, as is the nature of nursing.

The handbook is designed so that you can utilise individual chapters as a quick source of reference. Along with the activities and further recommended reading, it may also serve as a starting point for more in-depth study. Where website addresses are identified, these are only suggested sources of further information and others may be found through general search engines such as **www.google.co.uk**

The information offered relates mainly to health care in England, but we refer to Scotland, Wales and Northern Ireland when appropriate.

In writing this handbook we would like to acknowledge the support and assistance of all the Overseas Nurses Programme team, and of other colleagues at Bournemouth University.

Wendy Benbow
Gill Jordan

AUTHOR BIOGRAPHIES

Wendy Benbow

Following qualification as a registered nurse in 1969, Wendy worked for two years in genito-urinary surgery and major spinal injuries before moving into community nursing. Over a 14-year period Wendy was involved in a variety of roles that included community nursing sister, practice work teacher and nurse manager, as well as time seconded for research into leg ulcer care and co-ordinating pre-registration student placements for the local acute hospital.

After a year out to complete her teaching qualification, Wendy moved into full-time nurse education in 1985. Since then, she has been involved in both teaching and managing a range of pre- and post-registration courses, programme and curricular development, regionally-funded research and national project development. Most recently, Wendy has been involved in the development of student clinical placements in the care-home environment for pre-registration students and curricular development for post-qualified staff. Wendy is also link tutor to the local FE colleges for the Health and Social Care Foundation Degree and joint programme leader for the Overseas Nursing Programme.

Gill Jordan

On qualifying as a registered nurse in 1978, Gill completed her Orthopaedic Nursing Certificate and moved to New Zealand, where she worked in a large orthopaedic teaching hospital, ultimately as a ward sister of a trauma orthopaedic ward.

On her return to the UK in 1988, Gill moved into nurse education. Since then, she has been involved in a variety of courses and professional development programmes, both as a teacher and as a programme leader. These have included courses leading to professional registration, Return to Practice, Conversion Courses and various post-registration undergraduate programmes. Most recently, Gill has been involved in the Overseas Nursing Programme as joint programme leader.

Chapter 1

The Provision of Health Care in the UK

Changes to the provision and delivery of health care in the United Kingdom (UK), particularly since the early 1980s, have been, and still are, rapid and ongoing. This brief introduction to organisation and policy therefore seeks only to act as a useful starting-point for developing a more detailed understanding of how the system works.

Outcomes

On completion of this chapter you should be able to:

- identify the main structure and organisation of health and social care provision in the United Kingdom;

- outline the roles and responsibilities of the main organisations in the National Health Service and the independent sector;

- understand the key aims and strategies of current government policy;

- appreciate the similarities and differences between health care provision in the UK and the country where you completed your professional nurse education/training.

INTRODUCTION

The UK can be identified as a welfare state, a concept that refers to the state's provision of public measures and support for those in need across society (**www.lse.ac.uk**). Although the state's role in welfare began in the early years of the twentieth century, it was not until after the Second World War that the foundations of the current welfare state were fully established. Measures that were adopted at that time included policy and legislation to deal with what were known then as the interrelated 'Five Giants of Evil': want (poverty); ignorance (poor education); squalor (lack of and poor housing and town planning); idleness (unemployment) and disease (ill health). The specific policy utilised to combat disease and ill health was the introduction of a National Health Service (NHS). Today, despite many reorganisations and changes, health care in the United Kingdom is still mainly provided through the NHS, although the independent (or private) sector and the voluntary sector are increasingly becoming important partners in the overall provision.

THE NATIONAL HEALTH SERVICE (NHS)

Most formal care in the UK is provided by the NHS. It was established in 1948 (as part of a welfare state) as a free, comprehensive and universally co-ordinated health care service, available to the population as a whole. The original structure and organisation lasted until 1974, when the first major changes were made. Since then, in an effort to improve the quality and effectiveness of service provision, considerable and frequent change has taken place. In particular, the service has moved from being centrally directed and organised towards local decision making, providing a more client-focused service while creating, in theory, greater patient choice. Changes have and are also being implemented that seek to allow local communities greater influence and say over how their local services are run and delivered.

Today the NHS is a large and complex organisation covering many different services, each of which has different characteristics, different categories of staff and is provided through a variety of organisations. Advances in technology, a growing elderly population, higher expectations and greater knowledge have all increased the demands for health care, which have to be met out of a limited budget.

However, for all services, the government identifies five key objectives:

1 improve health and well being and reduce health inequalities and social exclusion;
2 secure access to a comprehensive range of services;
3 improve the quality, effectiveness and efficiency of services;
4 increase choice for patients and ensure a better experience of care through greater responsiveness to people's needs;
5 achieve best value within the resources provided.

(Department of Health, 2006a)

The service is still paid for mainly out of general taxation and, with the exception of some dental and optical care and prescribed drugs, it remains free at the point of delivery.

NHS ORGANISATION AND STRUCTURE

Prior to 1998 the NHS was organised and managed in the same way across England, Wales, Scotland and Northern Ireland. However, following devolution there has been an increasing divergence in both policy and structure within each of these countries. Although each country will be reviewed individually, the main focus for the chapter will centre on organisation and management for England.

ENGLAND

Activity

Note down the structure and key features of the health care system in which you completed your professional nurse education and training. Then take a few minutes to consider the diagram of the structure and organisation of the NHS in England in Figure 1.

Figure 1 explained

The Department of Health

The Department of Health supports the government in improving the health and well being of the population. The department provides strategic leadership to the NHS and social care organisations, including:

- setting overall direction;
- ensuring national standards are met;
- securing resources;
- making major investment decisions;
- improving choice for patients and users;
- improving standards of public health.

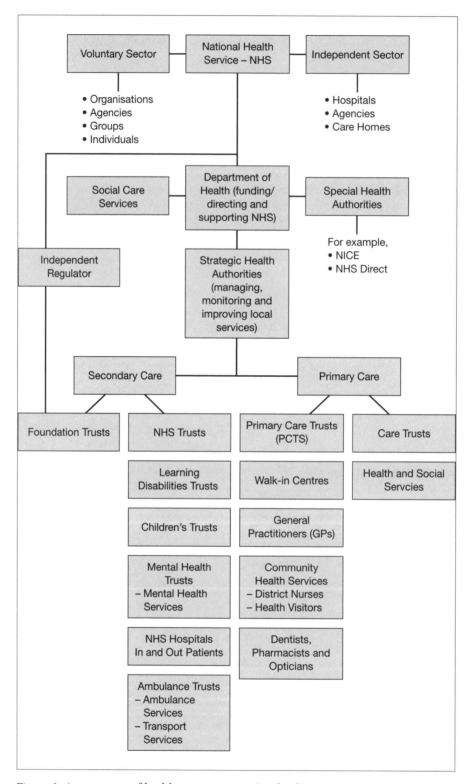

Figure 1 An overview of health care provision (England)

Strategic Health Authorities

Below the Department of Health there are now, following reconfiguration in July 2006, ten Strategic Health Authorities. The Strategic Health Authorities manage the NHS locally and are the key link between the Department of Health and the NHS. They are charged with:

- ensuring that national priorities are integrated into plans for the local health service;
- increasing the capacity of local health services to enable more services to be provided;
- monitoring the quality and performance of local health services;
- developing plans for improvement of health services in their local area.

Primary care

The term 'primary care' relates to community-based health services that are usually the first and, for some, the only point of contact that patients may have with the health service. It covers services provided by general practitioners (GPs), community and practice nurses, midwives, community therapists (e.g. physiotherapists and occupational therapists), community pharmacists, dentists and optometrists. NHS walk-in centres are also considered as part of primary care. While primary care is mostly concerned with patients' general health needs, more specialist treatments and services are becoming available in primary care settings closer to where people live.

Primary Care Trusts (PCTs)

Primary Care Trusts (PCTs) might now be considered the cornerstone of the NHS as they are viewed as taking the lead in the local health care system, and in England receive approximately 75–80 per cent of the NHS budget (Department of Health, 2006a). They currently have three main functions:

1 engaging with their local population to improve health and well being (in partnership with their Local Authority), including assessing the health needs of all the people in their local area and directly listening to patients' views on services;
2 commissioning a comprehensive and equitable range of high quality responsive and efficient services within allocated resources (these may include services from NHS Trusts, Foundation Trusts, independent hospitals or voluntary services and be from within the UK or from other European countries);
3 monitoring the quality and effectiveness of the services they provide.

Primary Care Trusts are accountable directly to their local population and to their Strategic Health Authority.

Care Trusts

Care Trusts were introduced in an attempt to enable closer integration between the health and social care sectors. They can be established when NHS organisations and Local Authorities agree to work in partnership to deliver services. To date only a few Care Trusts have been established.

NHS walk-in centres

Walk-in centres give fast access to health advice and treatment for minor illnesses and injuries. The centres are mostly nurse-led units and no appointment is necessary to access the service. Most are open seven days a week from early to late although a few provide a 24-hour service. They offer a variety of services that may include:

- assessment by a qualified nurse;
- treatment for minor illnesses and for minor injuries;
- advice on health promotion;
- information on other health services.

Many of these walk-in centres are now being developed by private companies but remain subject to the same quality monitoring as the NHS. **www.nhsdirect.nhs.uk**

Secondary care

The term 'secondary care' relates generally to acute hospital and specialist services, the funding of which now comes mainly from the Primary Care Trusts for commissioned services.

NHS Trusts

NHS Trusts employ the majority of the health service workforce in the UK. Trusts are largely self-governing but are accountable to the Strategic Health Authority for their performance management and to Primary Care Trusts for quality of commissioned health service provision and delivery.

Foundation Trusts

Relatively recently introduced, Foundation Trusts are organisations within the NHS that have greater freedom to develop and improve services at a local level and in response to local need. They are seen by the government as at the forefront of their commitment to the decentralisation of public services and the creation of a patient-led NHS. They are organised as separate entities and are deemed 'public benefit corporations', i.e. they are non-profit-making organisations and are perceived to be owned by their members, who are local people, employees and key stakeholders.

Foundation Trusts are not governed by the Department of Health (thereby, in theory, allowed more freedom) but are accountable to, and must adhere to arrangements made by an independent regulator who is accountable to Parliament. However, Foundation Trusts are still firmly part of the NHS and are thus still subject to NHS standards, performance ratings and systems of inspection through the Health Care Commission and through service-level agreements with PCTs and other NHS Trusts.

Special Health Authorities

These have been established to provide a 'national service' to the NHS. They are independent but can be subjected to ministerial direction like any other NHS body. They include, for example, the National Institute for Clinical Excellence (NICE) and NHS Direct.

National Institute for Health and Clinical Excellence (NICE)

Established in 2004, NICE was set up as an independent organisation whose overall remit is to bring together knowledge and guidance on ways of promoting good health and treating ill health. Guidance is developed using the expertise of the NHS and wider health care community including NHS staff, health care professionals, patients and carers, industry and the academic world.

NICE produces four kinds of guidance:

- *technology appraisals* – guidance on the use of new and existing medicines and treatments within the NHS in England and Wales;
- *clinical guidelines* – guidance on the appropriate treatment and care of people with specific diseases and conditions within the NHS in England and Wales;
- *interventional procedures* – guidance on whether interventional procedures used for diagnosis or treatment are safe enough and work well enough for routine use in England, Wales and Scotland;
- *promotion of good health and prevention of ill health*
  - public health intervention guidance – recommendations on locally delivered activities to reduce people's risk of illness or to promote healthy lifestyles;
  - public health programme guidance – recommended strategies, policies and multi-level action to improve health and reduce inequalities.

www.nice.org.uk

NHS Direct

NHS Direct is perceived by the government as playing a key role in the delivery to patients and the public of 24-hour health advice and information on a range of subjects (for example, self-care and access to local services). The service provides:

- an established telephone service (0845 4647);
- an online website (**www.nhsdirect.nhs.uk**);
- NHS Direct Interactive – an interactive public service on digital TV;
- a self-help guide delivered to homes across the UK.

Development of clinical services

Over the last 25 years, successive governments have produced a plethora of policy documents relating to the development of clinical services within the NHS. One such document which is of significant importance and, therefore, will briefly be considered here is *The NHS Plan: A Plan for Investment, a Plan for Reform*, published in July 2000 (Department of Health, 2000a).

The NHS Plan: A Plan for Investment, a Plan for Reform (2000)

Described by the government as the biggest change in health care since the NHS was formed in 1948, this ten-year plan outlined a range of targets and initiatives, some of which were new and some of which reflected earlier commitments. The overall emphasis of the plan was on investment and reform.

The key aspects of the plan were as follows:

- it identified that there would be no changes to the way the NHS was funded but that funding would be increased;
- it proposed increases in hospitals, bed capacity, equipment, consultants, GPs, nurses and other health care professionals;
- it gave a commitment to reducing the major causes of mortality and morbidity through the reduction of health inequalities;
- it proposed improving patient access to primary care and improving out patient/in patient and accident and emergency waiting times;
- it proposed expansion of intermediate care facilities, diagnostic and treatment centres, day surgery and short-stay treatment;
- it proposed improving joint working between the NHS and other care providers and identified the need to develop a greater role for the private (independent) sector;
- it identified a new performance-management system in which Trusts that were judged to have performed well could earn more autonomy on finances and service improvement;

- it proposed the setting of new national standards and creating a framework to support the delivery of those standards;
- it identified changes to the professions, including new contracts for consultants and GPs, a commitment to give nurses new roles and responsibilities, and improvements in professional regulation;
- it gave a commitment to improve collaboration and teamwork between different professions;
- it put forward plans to involve patients and the public at all levels of service provision;
- it gave commitments to improving public health.

(Department of Health, 2000a)

A number of these targets and initiatives have already been put into place by the government and you will recognise these within your employment as a qualified nurse.

Activity

Several further policy documents linked to *The NHS Plan* have been published. These include:

- The Health and Social Care (Community Health Standards) Bill (2003);
- *The NHS Improvement Plan: Putting People at the Heart of Public Services* (2004);
- *Making Partnerships Work for Patients, Carers and Service Users* (2004);
- *Creating a Patient-Led NHS* (2005);
- *Health Reforms in England: Update and Next Steps* (2005);
- *Health Reform in England: Update and Commissioning Framework* (2006);
- *Our Health, Our Care, Our Say: A New Direction for Community Services* (2006).

Executive summaries for all of the above can be accessed from **www.dh.gov.uk** and a review of these will provide you with a greater understanding of the current and future developments related to health care provision.

Clinical aspects of care

This area will be looked at in more detail as you work through this handbook. However, one long-term government policy launched in 1998 that can be considered here is the National Service Frameworks (NSFs) strategy.

National Service Frameworks (NSFs)

These frameworks form one of a range of measures that seek to raise quality and decrease variations in service across the NHS. (Variations in service are often referred to as the 'postcode lottery'.)

The government strategy through the NSFs so far published has been to:

- set national standards and define the way in which a service should be provided;
- put into practice strategies to support implementation;
- establish performance milestones against which progress within an agreed time scale can be measured.

Each NSF is developed with the assistance of an external reference group that involves health care professionals, service users and carers, health service managers, partner agencies and other advocates. The NSFs established to date are:

- Mental Health (1999);
- Paediatric Intensive Care (1999);
- Coronary Heart Disease (2000);
- Cancer (2000);
- Older People (2001);
- Diabetes (2001);
- Renal (2004);
- Children (2004);
- Long Term Conditions (2005);
- Chronic Obstructive Pulmonary Disease (COPD) (due to be published in 2008).

www.dh.gov.uk/en/Policyandguidance

NSFs are relevant to all providers and all deliverers of health care (particularly nurses) in England. Wales has embraced broadly similar frameworks while Scotland and Ireland have their own systems of clinical guidelines and service standards.

Activity

Given the importance of the NSFs, you should find it useful to review any of the above that are most likely to link to your proposed area of work. Further information on each of them can be accessed from **www.dh.gov.uk** Just type 'National Service Frameworks' in the search box.

WALES

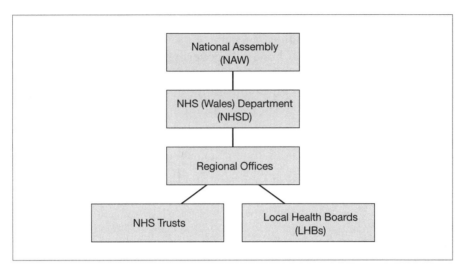

Figure 2 Overview of the structure of the NHS in Wales

Figure 2 explained

The National Assembly (NAW)

The NAW has full legislative power for health in Wales. It contains the Office of the Chief Medical Officer (who advises the government on health matters) and the Health and Social Services Committee (that contributes to Assembly policy development). The Welsh Assembly Government is the executive body of the NAW and includes the Minister for Health and Social Services. All NHS statutory organisations in Wales (including the Trusts and Local Health Boards) are accountable to the Minister for their performance and the Minister is ultimately accountable to the government for the overall running of the Welsh NHS. The Welsh Assembly Government is responsible for policy direction and dissemination of funds to the health service.

NHS (Wales) Department (NHSD)

The NHSD is an organisational arm of the Welsh Assembly Government, responsible for implementing the Assembly's policies and strategies for the management and development of the NHS in Wales. It is led by a Director and provides strategic leadership, as well as ensuring policy implementation. The department also advises the Minister for Health and Social Services about securing and allocating health resources, and monitors the performance of Local Health Boards and NHS Trusts.

Local Health Boards (LHBs)

Local Health Boards were created to bring greater accountability to the health service in Wales. They provide a simplified system for patients to understand while also enabling the service users to have a greater representative voice and say on how it is governed. The Health Boards are allocated 75 per cent of the overall budget for the NHS of Wales, and are therefore the main bodies to whom resources have been allocated for commissioning health care. Their responsibilities include:

- commissioning primary, community, and intermediate and secondary care services;
- assessing the health needs of their area and the effectiveness of the local health system.

NHS Trusts

NHS Trusts continue to run hospitals and provide secondary and specialist care. They also provide community services as there are no Primary Care Trusts in Wales.

(Royal College of General Practitioners, 2004)

Further information regarding the structure and work of the NHS in Wales can be obtained from **www.wales.nhs.uk**

Policy

In 2001 *Improving Health in Wales* (Welsh Assembly Government, 2001 – the Welsh equivalent of the *NHS Plan* in England) was launched. The document is available from **www.wales.nhs.uk/publications/primcare_e.pdf** and details a ten-year initiative to develop and improve health services in Wales. This includes the development and implementation of the National Service Frameworks (NSFs). Wales also embraces guidance from the National Institute for Health and Clinical Services (NICE).

SCOTLAND

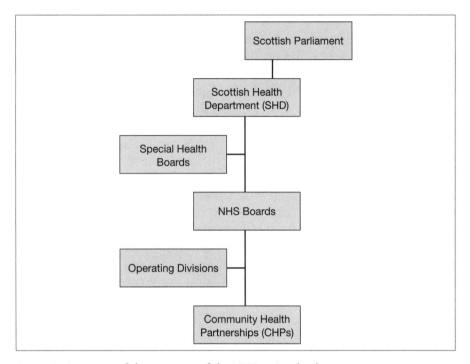

Figure 3 Overview of the structure of the NHS in Scotland

Figure 3 explained

The Scottish Parliament

The Scottish Parliament has full legislative power for health in Scotland. The Minister for Health and Community Care is accountable to the government for all health policies and the running of the NHS.

The Scottish Health Department (SHD)

This department is responsible for producing health policies and administering the NHS in Scotland.

Special Health Boards

The Special Health Boards provide services across the country and include NHS24, NHS Quality Improvement Scotland and the Scottish Ambulance Service.

NHS Boards

NHS Boards were created to:

- manage local health care organisations;
- give strategic direction and provide clinical governance.

They are also responsible for allocating funds and developing local health plans in association with local hospitals, GPs and NHS bodies.

Operating Divisions

Following the abolition of NHS Trusts and Primary Care Trusts in Scotland in 2004, operational management was transferred to Operating Divisions within the NHS Boards. There are a number of divisions within each Board and these allocate financial and decision-making powers to the appropriate organisations within their local health care system.

Operating Divisions for Primary Care within the Boards have taken over the responsibilities of the Primary Care Trusts. In particular they support general practice in the delivery of its services, give strategic direction and steer service improvement. They also oversee joint agreements between primary and secondary care clinicians on the design and delivery of services using joint investment funding.

Operating Divisions for Secondary Care have operational management responsibilities for running hospital services. These functions are devolved under standing orders from the NHS Board.

Community Health Partnerships (CHPs)

Community Health Partnerships (CHPs) are joint organisations comprising Local Authorities, and groups of GPs and other health professionals, in a defined geographic area. The aim of these partnerships is to integrate health services at a local level. Each partnership has a budget to develop and manage its own local priorities, deliver the NHS plan and to improve health care in the local communities.

(Royal College of General Practitioners, 2004)

> Further information regarding the structure and work of the NHS in Scotland can be accessed from:
>
> - www.scottish.parliament.uk/business/research/pdf_subj_maps/ smda-08.pdf
> - www.scotland.gov.uk
> - www.sehd.scot.nhs.uk/nationalframework/Reports.htm

Policy

In 2000 *Our National Health* (Scottish Executive, 2000 – the Scottish equivalent to *The NHS Plan* in England) was launched (available from **www.scotland.gov.uk**).

The National Institute for Health and Clinical Excellence (NICE) does not have a remit in Scotland. Instead, in 2003 a body called NHS Quality Improvement in Scotland was created to provide advice on good practice, set national standards and publish reports on NHS Scotland's performance (available from **www.nhshealthquality.org/nhsqis/CCC_FirstPage.jsp**).

In Scotland, NHS24 provides a service similar to that of NHS Direct and can be accessed on 084542 242424 or at **www.nhs24.com**

NORTHERN IRELAND

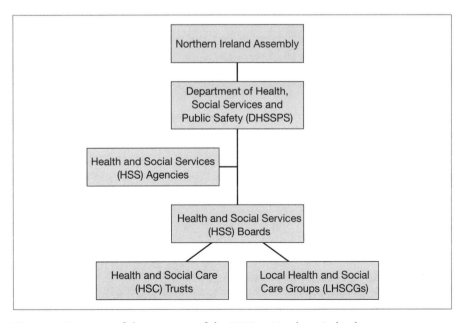

Figure 4 Overview of the structure of the NHS in Northern Ireland

Figure 4 explained

The Northern Ireland Assembly

On 14 October 2002 the Northern Ireland Assembly and Executive were suspended and responsibility for Health and Personal Social Services (HPSS) moved to the Northern Ireland Office. Devolved government was restored to the Assembly on 8 May 2007.

Department of Health, Social Services and Public Safety (DHSSPS)

The DHSSPS is responsible for creating policy and legislation for primary, secondary, community and social care, while also protecting and promoting public health and safety.

Health and Social Services (HSS) Agencies

The HSS Agencies provide services across the region and include the Health Promotion Agency and the Blood Transfusion Agency.

Health and Social Services (HSS) Boards

The HSS Boards act on behalf of the DHSSPS, assessing the local population and taking on the planning, commissioning and purchasing of health services.

Health and Social Services (HSS) Trusts

There are currently 19 HSS Trusts in Northern Ireland and all are directly accountable to the DHSSPS. They deliver the services commissioned by the HSS Boards. Seven of the Trusts deliver acute hospital services, five deliver community health and social care services, and six provide both hospital and community care. One Trust deals with the provision of ambulance services.

Local Health and Social Care Groups (LHSCGs)

These are committees of their local HSS Boards and their role is to plan and develop primary care services. They are involved in commissioning decisions and receive a budget for this purpose.

(Royal College of General Practitioners, 2004)

> Further information on the structure and the way in which the NHS works in Northern Ireland can be obtained from **www.healthand careni.co.uk**

Policy

In 2000 *Investing in Health* (a document equivalent to *The NHS Plan* in England) was launched (available from **www.investingforhealthni.gov.uk**). Plans for restructuring the NHS in Northern Ireland were on hold during the suspension of the Northern Ireland Assembly.

The National Institute for Health and Clinical Excellence (NICE) does not have a remit in Northern Ireland and NHS Direct is the same as for England. In Northern Ireland, unlike England, Wales and Scotland, health and social services have been integrated as one system since 1972.

SUMMARY OF THE STRUCTURE AND ORGANISATION OF THE NHS IN THE UK

The structure and organisation of the NHS does differ within the UK. However, the overriding principle of the NHS being a free and comprehensive health service available to the population as a whole remains the same.

Organisation	England	Wales	Scotland	N. Ireland
Government department	Department of Health	NHSD	SHD	DHSSPS
Strategic direction	Stategic Health Authorities	Regional Offices	NHS Boards	HSS Boards
Primary care management	PCTs	LHBs	Operating Division for Primary Care	LHSCGs
Hospital management	NHS Trusts	NHS Trusts	Operating Division for Secondary Care	HSS Trusts
Community care management	PCTs and NHS Trusts	NHS Trusts	Operating Divisions	HSS Trusts
Social Services Management	Local Authorities	Local Authorities and LHBs	SHD and Local Authorities	HSS Trusts

Figure 5 A summary of the structure and organisation of the NHS in the UK (Royal College of General Practitioners, 2004)

THE INDEPENDENT SECTOR (PRIVATE SECTOR)

According to Baggot (2004) it is difficult to estimate fully the size of the independent sector within the UK, owing mainly to its diversity. It consists of large and small private organisations as well as individual practitioners working partly or wholly in a private capacity. It also includes a considerable range of health care services, from acute hospitals and nursing homes through to dentistry and alternative medicine. What further complicates the issue is that patients may also pay privately for some NHS services (for example, treatment in an NHS hospital). In fact, according to Laing and Buisson (2001), the NHS was the largest single supplier of private treatment and acute health care in the UK, with a market share at that time of approximately 14 per cent.

While the health care system is still predominately a public service model, it is clear that, overall, the independent sector has become increasingly important over the past three decades in the provision and delivery of health care services.

Baggott identifies that in 2000 the government sought to improve collaboration by formulating an agreement with the independent sector (Independent Health Care Association and Department of Health, 2000), which was intended as an enabling framework to foster closer involvement of the independent sector in:

- planning, commissioning or subcontracting of services from it in order to expand the capacity of the health care system;
- closer co-operation in workforce planning;
- the provision of information on adverse clinical effects, clinical performance and treatment of NHS patients.

(Baggot, 2004, p. 153)

The independent sector continues to be viewed by the government as an important partner to the NHS in the quest to deliver more convenient care and choice to NHS patients.

Private health insurance

Although successive governments have actively encouraged the take up of personal private health insurance the majority of private health insurance schemes (approximately 66 per cent) are organised by employers and the uptake has remained relatively low and stable over the past decade (Baggot, 2004).

Starting points for further information regarding the independent sector can be obtained from:

- www.hd.gov.uk
- www.independenthealthcare.org.uk

THE VOLUNTARY CARE SECTOR (VCS)

The voluntary care sector (VCS) has a long tradition in the UK of providing services directly to the community and to specific client groups, particularly those who fall outside the so-called mainstream health and social care system. As elsewhere, voluntary organisations in the UK range from international organisations with professional staff (for example, the Red Cross), to national organisations (for example, the Multiple Sclerosis Society) and small local groups that operate on a largely informal basis.

As with the independent sector, there has been a significant move towards including the VCS in the provision and delivery of health care within the UK. In 2004 representatives from the VCS, health and social care and the Department of Health reviewed ways to promote further the increasing role of the voluntary sector through contributions to health service planning and delivery. There followed a jointly-developed agreement between the government, the NHS and the VCS that established a framework of partnership working through the introduction of the National Strategic Partnership Forum (NSPF).

The NSPF is a departmental working group of the Department of Health and reports to ministers. Its membership consists of individuals representing organisations from the VCS, NHS and social care, local government and the Department of Health. The primary principle underpinning the purpose and work of the Forum is a commitment to improving the experience of patients, service users and carers by helping the voluntary, community and public services to work more effectively together.

(Department of Health, 2005)

Activity

Using a general search engine such as **www.google.co.uk** or other information services such as the local library, identify further examples of international, national and locally-based voluntary care groups that support the delivery and provision of health care within the UK.

SOCIAL CARE

Social care in the UK is another of the major public service areas. In England the responsibility to provide social care services rests principally with Local Authorities (councils). Since the 1980s there have been numerous government initiatives to integrate more closely the provision and delivery of social and health care, including the introduction of Care Trusts. Providers of social care are now expected to work closely with others including the NHS, voluntary and independent organisations as well as the education service, the probation service, the police and other agencies who share the responsibility to provide social care and support.

Social care services may be offered in a variety of settings including hospitals, health centres, educational settings, community groups, residential homes, advice centres and in people's own homes. There are a considerable number of social care services available in most local authorities and these may include:

- adoption;
- Aids and HIV;
- carers;
- child protection;
- children in care;
- community development;
- day care;
- elderly people;
- families;
- fostering;
- home adaptations;
- home help;
- learning disabilities;
- leaving hospital;
- mental health;
- care homes;
- personal care at home;
- residential care;
- respite care;
- substance misuse;
- voluntary organisations.

Regulation and monitoring

The Commission for Social Care Inspection (CSCI) provides independent monitoring, regarding both the quality and performance of the whole social care sector, for the government and public (a brief overview of the Commission's work can be found in Chapter 4, page 74).

Further information regarding the provision of social care within the UK can be accessed from:

- www.dh.gov.uk
- www.nhs.uk
- www.dh.gov.uk/en/Publicationsandstatistics/Publications/
  Publications PolicyAndGuidance/DH_074217

The last site provides a review of the current (2007) arrangements for promoting the contribution that social care makes to the provision of people's independence, inclusion, health and well being. It also makes recommendations for further development in the service.

Activity

Having briefly explored the provision of health care in the UK, review your notes from the first activity in this chapter (page 3) and make notes on the similarities and differences between provision here and in the country where you completed your nurse education/training programme.

Useful websites

- www.nhsdirect.nhs.uk
- www.dh.gov.uk/en/Policyandguidance

Chapter 2

Legal, Professional and Ethical Issues

The aim of this chapter is to make you aware of the legal and professional issues surrounding nursing in the UK. There is also a section on ethics; the information in which may not be new to you, but should be viewed in conjunction with the legal and professional aspects of nursing.

Outcomes

On completion of this chapter you should be able to:

- demonstrate an awareness of the legal system in the UK;

- discuss the legal responsibilities of a registered nurse when caring for patients or clients;

- define the term 'accountability' in relation to the *Code of Professional Conduct: Standards for Conduct, Performance and Ethics* (NMC, 2004a) and other guidelines issued by the Nursing and Midwifery Council;

- discuss the principles of health care ethics and relate their use to situations in clinical practice.

ACCOUNTABILITY

'To be accountable is literally to be liable to be called upon to give an account of what one has done or not done' (Banks, 2004, p. 150). The importance of accountability in professional life is not new, but there is an increasing focus on issues surrounding accountability and nurses must be aware of the implications it brings.

Accountability is often defined as responsibility, but there is a difference between the two. Responsibility is concerned with answering for what you do, whereas accountability is being answerable for the *consequences* of what you do. The most important factor in accountability is that it is 'personal' and no other practitioner can be accountable for another. The Nursing and Midwifery Council (NMC, 2004a, p. 4) states this very clearly in its *Code of Professional Practice* (clause 1.3):

> You are personally accountable for your practice. This means that you are answerable for your actions and omissions, regardless of advice or directions from another professional.

Castledine (1991, p. 28) offers a further definition of accountability and, although written some time ago, it is still very pertinent today as it encompasses the whole ethos of how accountability in nursing should be viewed. He states that accountability is:

> that phenomena related to nursing practice which nurses are entrusted with, are answerable for, take the credit and the blame for, and can be judged within legal and moral boundaries.

Arenas of accountability

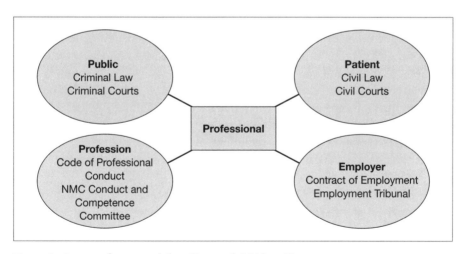

Figure 1 Arenas of accountability (Dimond, 2005, p. 5)

Criminal law

A crime is committed against the state either when an act is performed which the law forbids, or when an act is omitted which the law requires.

For a conviction it must be proved that a person intended to commit the crime, or was reckless in doing the criminal act. More serious cases include murder, manslaughter and rape (all of which nurses have been found guilty) and these are heard in Crown Courts before a judge and jury. Lesser cases (for example, driving offences) are heard in a magistrate's court. The outcome of prosecution may be a custodial sentence or fine.

Civil law

This part of the law involves the rights and duties individuals have towards each other. Legal action can be taken by a private individual against another individual or an organisation. This is the main legal area which affects nurses and which lawyers refer to as the Law of Torts. The outcomes from these actions, if successful, usually involve awards of compensation (for damages) or orders (injunctions) to stop an individual acting unlawfully. It is interesting to note that the NMC recognises that this is an area in which nurses are increasingly involved and, in the 2004 version of its *Code of Professional Conduct: Standards for Conduct, Performance and Ethics*, it has added a clause in which it recommends nurses have professional indemnity insurance – 'in the event of claims of professional negligence' (NMC, 2004a, p. 11).

An action for negligence is a civil action, and results from a breach of the duty of care. A nurse may be held legally liable if it can be shown either that they have failed to exercise the skills properly expected of them, or that they have undertaken tasks that they are not competent to perform (Dimond, 2005). For negligence to be proved three conditions must be satisfied:

1 that a duty of care was owed by the defendant (nurse) to the plaintiff (patient) – the nurse/patient relationship;
2 that there was a breach in the standard of care;
3 that this breach has caused harm either by action or by omission.

Some defendants in criminal cases may also have a civil action brought against them if any harm has been caused by 'action or omission'.

Activity

- Think of a circumstance where you, as a registered nurse, might be held criminally liable.
- Describe three circumstances in clinical practice where you may be judged negligent.

Accountability to the employer

All practitioners are accountable to their employer. There is an implied term in every contract of employment that the employee will obey the reasonable instructions of the employer (that is, follow any policies, procedures, standards, etc.), and that any employee who breaches their contract may be subject to disciplinary action.

An employer is liable for civil actions (torts) committed by their employees (for example, nurses) during the scope of their employment. This is called 'vicarious liability' but does not remove any legal responsibility from the employee, as vicarious liability is an additional liability not a substituted one. The employer (for example, a NHS Trust or care home) cannot delegate their duty by saying that they provide competent trained staff. They will always be primarily responsible for any negligence to patients.

However, if a patient takes out an action against an employer, and the employer is found directly liable because of harm caused by an employee, the employer could take out an action against that individual employee. This usually happens when an employer has to pay compensation to a patient as a result of an employee's negligence, and tries to recoup their money from the employee.

Professional liability

The NMC emphasises the need for practitioners to be accountable for their practice by issuing the *Code of Professional Conduct: Standards for Conduct, Performance and Ethics* (NMC, 2004a) to all its practitioners. Although this document is not part of law (Burnard and Chapman, 2003), the functions of the NMC include a requirement to establish and improve standards of training and professional conduct (Nursing and Midwifery Order, 2001), and it does this by issuing the Code and a requirement for all practitioners to abide by it. Therefore, the Code acts as a reminder of the standards required by the profession. Breaching the *Code of Professional Conduct* is in effect a breach of registration and may lead to the removal of the nurse's name from the register and, consequently, the right to practise (Peate, 2006).

Paramount in this document, along with the practitioner's need to be accountable for their practice, is the mandatory requirement to promote and safeguard the interests of patients and clients. In addition it states that all practitioners 'must keep knowledge, skills and abilities required for lawful, safe and effective practice' (NMC, 2004a, p. 9).

Further to the *Code of Professional Conduct*, the NMC issues *Guidelines for the Administration of Medicines* (2004b), *Guidelines for Records and Record-Keeping* (2005) and *The PREP (Post-Registration Education and Practice Handbook)* (2006a) to all practitioners. While, again, these have no legal force in themselves, their recommendations are firm guidelines to all practitioners who require clear evidence to justify any actions.

See also the section on the NMC pages 26–28.

Summarising accountability

Each registered nurse must ensure that they fulfil their duties according to the approved standards of practice expected of them. If something goes wrong they are accountable in the criminal courts, in the civil courts, before their employer and before the Fitness to Practice Committee of the NMC for their activities, and would have to show that they had followed the approved accepted practice (Dimond, 2005).

This section has given a very brief introduction to the law in the UK. Further detail can be found in a variety of texts written for nurses, perhaps the most comprehensive being Bridgit Dimond's *Legal Aspects of Nursing* and Helen Caulfield's *Vital Notes for Nurses: Accountability* (see References, page 181).

THE NURSING AND MIDWIFERY COUNCIL (NMC)

The NMC is an organisation set up by Parliament to protect the public by ensuring that nurses and midwives provide high standards of care to their patients and clients. To achieve its aims, the NMC:

- maintains a register of qualified nurses, midwives and specialist community public health nurses;
- sets standards for conduct, performance and ethics;
- provides advice for nurses and midwives;
- considers allegations of misconduct, lack of competence or unfitness to practise due to ill health.

Furthermore, the NMC, in issuing its *Code of Professional Conduct* (NMC, 2004a, p. 4) states that its duty is to:

- inform the profession of the standard of professional conduct required of them in the exercise of their professional accountability and practice;

- inform the public, other professions and employers of the standard of professional conduct they can expect of a registered practitioner.

The powers of the NMC are set out in the Nursing and Midwifery Order 2001, and include the power to remove or caution any practitioner who is found guilty of professional misconduct. In some cases (for example, practitioners charged with serious crimes) it can also suspend a registrant while the case is under investigation.

All nurses in the UK working in a registered nurse capacity must be registered with the NMC. The NMC has recently redesigned the parts of the register, the sections being as outlined below in Figure 2:

Registerable Qualifications – 1st Level Nurses – Sub-part 1

Adult

Mental Health

Learning Disabilities

Children

Recorded Qualifications:

Mode 1 Prescribing

Extended Nurse Prescribing

Extended/Supplementary Nursing Prescribing

Practice Teacher / Teacher

Specialist Practitioner – Adult Nursing

Specialist Practitioner – Mental Health

Specialist Practitioner – Children's Nursing

Specialist Practitioner – Learning Disability Nurse

Specialist Practitioner – General Practice Nursing

Specialist Practitioner – Community Mental Health Nursing

Specialist Practitioner – Community Learning Disabilities Nursing

Specialist Practitioner – Community Children's Nursing

Specialist Practitioner – Occupational Health Nursing

Specialist Practitioner – School Nursing

Specialist Practitioner – District Nursing

Figure 2 The structure of the NMC Register of Qualified Nurses (Dimond, 2005, p. 5)

Code of Professional Conduct

The Code is divided into sections, with an overall introduction that clearly states:

- you are personally accountable for your practice – this means that you are answerable for your actions and omissions, regardless of advice or directions from another professional;

- you have a duty of care to your patients and clients, who are entitled to receive safe and competent care;

- you must adhere to the laws of the country in which you are practising.

(NMC, 2004a, p. 4)

This sets the scene for the other sections and clauses, which are summarised thus. As a Registered Nurse you must:

- Protect and support the health of individual patients and clients;
- protect and support the health of the wider community;
- act in such a way that justifies the trust and confidence the public have in you;
- uphold and enhance the good reputation of the professions.

- Respect the patient or client as an individual;
- obtain consent before you give any treatment or care;
- co-operate with others in the team;
- protect confidential information.

- Maintain your professional knowledge and competence;
- be trustworthy;
- act to identify and minimise the risks to patients and clients.

(NMC, 2004a)

DELEGATION

Although the Code emphasises that all practitioners are personally accountable for their practice, there may be some instances where nurses may be delegated tasks, or indeed delegate tasks themselves. In these cases it is important to remember the legal perspective on this and, according to Peate (2006), the following must be borne in mind.

- When working as a team member you are personally accountable for your own actions or omissions – there is no such concept as team negligence. If harm occurs, you are individually accountable.
- You must determine if the person you are delegating to is able to undertake the task. You must provide them with adequate resources and supervision. They must be deemed competent.
- You must keep up to date your knowledge and skills in order to practise safely and effectively within the scope of the law. You must acknowledge your limitations.
- You must make known and obtain help and supervision from a competent practitioner if you feel an aspect of practice lies beyond your level of competence or outside your area of registration.

The following pages look at some of the issues the Code raises in more detail: issues of consent; confidentiality; record-keeping and maintaining professional knowledge and competence.

Case study

Read the following article and identify and comment on the six clauses of the *Code of Professional Conduct* (NMC, 2004a) that Jo breached. (Reproduced with permission from the *British Journal of Nursing.*)

STAFF NURSE WHO FAILED TO PROVIDE ADEQUATE NURSING CARE FOR PATIENTS

British Journal of Nursing, 2004, 13: 389: Professional Misconduct Series

In the following case a senior nurse called Jo deliberately ignored certain aspects of care while on night duty because she felt that it was not her responsibility to do certain tasks or check that they had been carried out.

Jo worked on nights for a large inner-city hospital trust and had been doing so for over 10 years. When working on the general medical/surgical wards she was often heard to say derogatory remarks about some of the patients or core nursing tasks she was expected to do. For example, she saw it as a junior nursing role to go round and attend to patients' pressure needs. She felt her expertise lay in giving out drugs, managing intravenous infusion lines and doing certain nursing procedures.

On the particular ward where she was working two patients requested pain relief. Jo did not bother to go and see the patients, but instructed two healthcare assistants who were on duty with her to give each of the patients two paracetamol tablets. The healthcare assistants gave the medication to the patients as directed, but at no time did Jo attempt to check what they had given or to clarify with the patients how they were feeling. The situation continued for several shifts. Any patient who required additional pain relief was referred by the healthcare assistants to Jo, who told them to give paracetamol.

On the last occasion that Jo and the healthcare assistants were on duty together, an agency nurse was also present because of the workload on the ward. However, Jo still did not help unless she felt it was absolutely necessary. At one time during the evening she left the ward for a break stating that she had left the keys on the shelf in the office. These keys included keys to the controlled drug cupboard and the drugs trolley. Although Jo was entitled to a break from the ward, this was the third she had taken that night and she did not tell the staff where she was going.

The agency nurse was angry that Jo had left the ward without informing her of where she was going and how she could be contacted. Jo also did not tell the agency nurse where she could find the keys. A patient then complained of pain and the healthcare assistant asked the agency nurse, who was a registered nurse, if she could give the patient some paracetamol. The agency nurse then questioned the healthcare assistants about the procedure they had been following with Jo.

When Jo eventually returned to the ward, the agency nurse challenged her about the drug administration and leaving the keys in the ward office. Jo was offhand with the agency nurse and did not speak to her for the rest of the shift. At the handover to the day staff, Jo gave the report without involving the rest of the night nursing team. She let the healthcare assistants and the agency nurse write up the nursing records, but at no time in the handover did she involve them in the verbal report.

The agency nurse complained to the ward manager about the incidents that had occurred, and also some problems relating to a blood transfusion that Jo had been managing. It appeared that Jo had not followed the trust protocol with regard to administration of a transfusion. There had been a long delay before it had been commenced and Jo had not recorded any observations of the patient during the transfusion.

An investigation was carried out by the trust and it was felt that Jo should be dismissed from her post and her case referred to the Nursing and Midwifery Council. Jo was charged by the NMC and found guilty of:

- failing to provide adequate support for patients on a ward
- giving medication to healthcare assistants to administer to patients

- leaving a ward without advising staff of her whereabouts, and not handing over the ward keys to a registered nurse colleague
- failing to provide an adequate and appropriate hand-over of patient care
- failing to follow the correct protocol and procedure while administering a blood transfusion

Her name was removed from the nursing register.

Note: this case is in a series based on actual true cases which were reported to the NMC. Complied by George Castledine, Professor and Consultant of General Nursing, University of Central England, Birmingham, and Dudley Group of Hospitals NHS Trust.

CONSENT

Any adult, mentally competent person has the right in law to consent to any touching of their person, or to refuse any examination or treatment. If they are touched without consent or other lawful justification, then the person has the right to bring a criminal action for battery, or a civil action for trespass to the person (Dimond, 2005). Furthermore, should harm occur to the patient it could result in a legal action against the nurse for negligence. Consent also affirms the person's right to self-determination and autonomy (Caulfield, 2005). Lord Donaldson points out that consent is twofold – first, to obtain 'legal' justification for care (as above), and secondly, 'clinical' consent to secure the patient's trust and co-operation.

Consent can be given in written or verbal form or is implied ('by co-operation'). They are all equally valid. However, these forms vary considerably in their value as evidence in proving that consent was given. Consent in writing is the best form of evidence and is therefore the preferred method of obtaining the consent of the patient when any procedure involving some risk is contemplated.

It must be remembered that it is a basic principle of law in the UK that an adult, mentally competent person has the right to refuse treatment and take their own discharge contrary to medical advice. The NMC (2004a, p. 5) endorses this by saying that: 'as a registered nurse … you must obtain consent before you give any treatment or care'. It also states that it is a professional duty that any information given to allow the patient to make an informed decision must be accurate, truthful and presented in such a way as to make it easily understood.

Therefore, consent must be:

- given by a legally competent person;
- informed;
- given freely.

A legally competent person

The person giving consent must have the capacity to do so. A legally competent person must be able to understand and retain treatment information and use the information to make an informed decision. It is presumed that a patient is competent unless otherwise assessed by a 'suitably qualified practitioner' (NMC, 2004a, p. 6). No-one has the right to consent on behalf of another competent adult. Further, it is accepted that adults over the age of 16 have the relevant capacity to understand and make their own decisions about medical and nursing treatment (Caulfield, 2005).

Informed consent

The patient must be able to give informed consent to the proposed treatments and the information, given by a health care professional, should include any material risks: for example, the nature and consequences of the proposed treatment, and the consequences of not having the treatment and any alternatives to the treatment.

Consent must be given freely

This means that no threats or implied threats must be used, that no 'coercion and undue influence' is applied. Coercion invalidates consent and, if a health care professional feels that the patient is being coerced, either by another health care professional or by family, they should seek to see the patient alone to ascertain that *their* wishes are being adhered to (Peate, 2006).

Children and young people

If the patient is under 18 years old (the age of consent) the rules concerning consent are different. A person aged 16–17 is allowed to consent to treatment under the Family Law Reform Act (1979), in a similar way to an adult. However, refusal of treatment can be overridden by a person with parental authority or a court order.

A person under the age of 16 years who has sufficient understanding and intelligence to enable them to understand the proposed treatment or investigation may have the capacity to consent (Department of Health, 2001a). Children who have these capacities are said to be 'Gillick competent' (Peate, 2006). The term 'Gillick' (sometimes referred to as 'Fraser' after the judge who heard the case) comes from a court case in 1985, which concerned a teenage girl's right to consent to medical treatment without her parent's knowledge (*Gillick* v. *West Norfolk and Wisbech Area Health Authority*). An assessment to determine whether a minor is Gillick competent must ask the following questions:

- Does the child understand the proposed treatment, his/her medical condition, and the consequences that may emerge if he/she refuses or agrees to treatment?
- Does he/she understand the moral, social and family issues involved in the decision he/she is to make?
- Does the mental state of the child fluctuate?
- What treatment is to be performed – does the child understand the complexities of the proposed treatment and the potential risks associated with it?

(Peate, 2006, p. 72)

Mental Capacity Act (2005)

The Mental Capacity Act, which was passed in 2005, became law in 2007 and affects people living in England and Wales over the age of 16. It is concerned with protecting people who lack capacity to make their own decisions about a variety of health and social circumstances. The Act introduces:

- a new test to determine 'a person's best interests';
- new Lasting Powers of Attorney which extend to a person's health and welfare as well as to their property and money;
- a new Court of Protection and a new office of Public Guardian to support the Court;
- deputies who can make decisions in a 'person's best interests';
- a new criminal offence of ill-treatment and neglect;
- regulation of advance decisions to refuse treatment;
- regulation of research in relation to individuals who lack mental capacity;
- a new Independent Mental Capacity Advocate service (IMCA) for people with no family or friends;
- a Code of Practice to accompany the Act – health care professionals will have a duty to abide by the Code.

The underlying principles of the Mental Capacity Act (2005) are as follows (see **www.ncpc.org.uk**).

- A presumption of capacity: everyone has the right to their own decisions, so a person must be assumed to have capacity unless it is established that they lack capacity.
- Individuals should be supported where possible so that they can make their own decisions: a person must not be treated as being unable to make a decision unless all practicable steps to help them to do so have been taken, without success.
- People have the right to make decisions which may seem eccentric or unwise to other people: a person is not to be treated as unable to make a clear decision merely because they make an unwise decision.
- Best interests: acts done or decisions made on behalf of a person established to be lacking capacity must be in their best interests.
- Rights and freedoms must be restricted as little as possible: before an act is done or a decision taken on behalf of a person, regard must be had as to whether the purpose underlying that act or decision can be achieved in a way less restrictive of their rights or freedom of action.
- A person who lacks capacity is unable to make a decision for themselves by reason of disturbance of their mind or brain, whether on a temporary or permanent basis.
- A person is unable to make a decision if they cannot understand relevant information, retain that information, use or weigh that information as part of making a decision, or is unable to communicate their decision 'by any means'.
- Lack of capacity cannot be established merely by reference to a person's age, appearance, or behaviour.

Adults who cannot consent

Some adults may not have the capacity to provide consent to treatment or care. Evaluation of their capacity is the key to deciding whether a person has lost capacity on a temporary or permanent basis, and it may be that where a patient refuses treatment that evaluation of capacity takes place. If a patient cannot consent then health professionals are obliged to treat them in accordance with 'their best interests' – including the whole assessment of their welfare. In 'their best interests' is said to be when a 'body of other similar treatment providers would also give the same treatment' (Tingle and Cribb, 2006, p. 168), and arises from a court case in 1989 (*F* v. *West Berkshire Health Authority*). Adults who are incapable of giving consent because of mental illness can receive treatment under the provisions of the Mental Health Act (1983).

Advanced decisions to refuse treatment

The Mental Capacity Act (2005) allows patients over the age of 18 years to state, in writing, in advance what treatment they would not like carried out should they become unable to decide for themselves, and this must be respected by health care professionals. The patient must be deemed competent when making the advanced directive, and only clear refusals of specific treatments will be upheld. If any doubt exists, then treatment may be given 'in the patient's best interests'. Furthermore, a patient cannot refuse basic care.

Further information about consent can be obtained from the Department of Health website at **www.dh.gov.uk** (type 'consent' into the main search engine). Key guidance includes:

- a reference guide to the principles of consent to examination and treatment;
- good practice in consent implementation guide.

In addition, on the same website there is information about consent forms and associated guidance for patients. Another website pertaining to the Mental Capacity Act (2005) is **www.dca.gov.uk** (type 'MCA' into the search engine).

CONFIDENTIALITY

Confidentiality is a fundamental part of the patient/client relationship. Any information given to a nurse by a patient should not be passed on to anyone outside the health care team without consent. The fundamental importance of trust between a health professional and the patient brings with it a 'duty of confidence' (Caulfield, 2005).

This duty arises from:

- duty of care in negligence (discussed earlier in the chapter, page 24) – a breach of confidentiality can lead to civil action;
- implied duties under the nurse's contract of employment;
- requirements of the NMC outlined in its *Code of Professional Conduct* (NMC, 2004a, p. 8) – a breach of this could result in removal from the nurses' register.

The NMC further endorses Caulfield's statements in its Code by stating: 'you must treat information about patients and clients as confidential and use it only for the purposes for which it was given' (NMC, 2004a, p. 8). Other legislation concerning confidentiality includes the following.

- The Data Protection Act 1998, which gives the patient a statutory right to access any personal information in the form of health records held on them (both computer and manually-held records). The definition of 'health record' includes all records relating to their health: for example, nursing records, physiotherapy records, laboratory results, etc. The patient also has the right of rectification (making right/amendment) if the data recorded appears to be inaccurate.
- The Access to Medical Reports Act 1988, which gives an individual the right of access to any medical report relating to them which has been supplied by a medical practitioner for employment purposes or insurance purposes (Dimond, 2005).
- Article 8 of the European Convention of Human Rights (1998), which enables individuals to bring actions against public authorities who have failed to uphold a person's right to respect for private and family life (Dimond, 2005).

Caldicott

A review was commissioned in 1997 by the Chief Medical Officer of England owing to:

> ... increasing concern about the ways in which patient information [was] being used in the NHS in England and Wales and the need to ensure that confidentiality [was] not undermined. Such concern was largely due to the development of information technology in the service, and its capacity to disseminate information about patients rapidly and extensively.
> (Department of Health, 1999a, p. 1)

As a result of the report every NHS organisation is required to appoint a 'Caldicott Guardian' who is responsible for agreeing and reviewing internal protocols governing the protection and use of patient-identifiable information by the staff of their organisation.

Summarising confidentiality

According to Dimond (2005) there are seven exceptions to the duty of confidence, when nurses can divulge information about their patients:

1 with the patient's consent;
2 in the patient's best interests;
3 as a result of a court order;
4 as a result of a statutory duty to disclose;
5 in the public's interests;
6 if asked to do so by the police;
7 under provisions within the Data Protection Act (1998).

Further information about confidentiality can be obtained from the Department of Health Website at **www.dh.gov.uk** (type 'confidentiality code of practice' into the main search engine). Key guidance includes:

- an introduction the concept of confidentiality;
- a description of what a confidential service should look like;
- provision of a high-level description of the main legal requirements;
- recommendations for a generic decision support tool for sharing/disclosing information;
- a list of examples of particular information disclosure scenarios.

RECORDS AND RECORD-KEEPING

Record-keeping is part of the professional duty of care owed by the nurse to the patient. The NMC states this in its *Guidelines for Records and Record-Keeping*:

> Record-keeping is an integral part of nursing and midwifery practice. It is a tool of professional practice and one that should help the care process. It is not separate from this process and it is not an optional extra to be fitted in if circumstances allow.
>
> (NMC, 2005a, p. 6)

The NMC (2005a) further says that good record-keeping helps to protect the welfare of patients and clients by promoting:

- high standards of clinical care;
- continuity of care;
- better communication and dissemination of information between members of the inter-professional health care team;
- an accurate account of treatment and care planning and delivery;
- the ability to detect problems, such as changes in the patient's or client's condition, at any stage.

Therefore, failure to maintain reasonable standards of record-keeping could be evidence of professional misconduct and subject to Fitness to Practice proceedings. All nurses should be familiar with the NMC guidelines, which can be accessed at **www.nmc-uk.org** The salient points are that patient/client records should:

- be factual, consistent and accurate;
- be written/electronically recorded as soon as possible after an event has occurred, providing current information on the care and condition of the patient/client;
- be written clearly and in such a manner that the text cannot be erased or deleted without a record of change;
- be written in such a manner that any justifiable alterations or additions are dated, timed and signed or clearly attributed to a named person in an identifiable role in such a way that the original entry can still be read clearly;
- be accurately dated, timed and signed, with the signature printed alongside the first entry where this is a written record, and attributed to a named person in an identifiable role for electronic records;
- not include abbreviations, jargon, meaningless phrases, irrelevant speculation and offensive subjective statements;
- be readable on any photocopies.

In addition, records should:

- be written, wherever possible, with the involvement of the patient/client or their carer;
- be written in terms that the patient/client can understand;
- be consecutive;
- identify problems that have arisen and the action taken to rectify them;
- provide clear evidence of the care planned, the decisions made, the care delivered and the information shared.

Accurate record-keeping is vital as records can be called as evidence by the Health Services Commissioner, before a court of law, or in a local investigation of a complaint made by a patient. The NMC may also request records when investigating complaints about nurses at Fitness to Practice hearings. These records may include anything that makes reference to a patient (for example, care plans, diaries, etc.), and any absence of a record may be seen as a lack of care, negligence, inability to write a record, disinterest, concealment or a general failure to communicate in the best interest of the patient. A coroner recently stated: 'Nurses are good observers – it's only a question of whether or not they write their observations down. When they come to court to testify, facts which seemed trivial at the time take on a paramount importance' (anon).

MAINTAINING PROFESSIONAL KNOWLEDGE AND COMPETENCE

Post-Registration Education and Practice (PREP) is a set of NMC professional standards and guidance (NMC, 2006a) that is designed to help nurses provide the best possible care for patients and clients. The fulfilment of PREP requirements helps nurses keep up to date with developments in practice and encourages thinking and reflection.

In order to renew registration nurses must provide a signed Notification of Practice (NOP) which asks them, among other things, to declare that they have met the PREP requirements. There are two separate PREP standards which affect registration (NMC, 2006a):

- The PREP Practice Standard – nurses must have worked in some capacity by virtue of their nursing, midwifery or specialist community public health nursing qualification a minimum of 450 hours during the previous three years, or have successfully undertaken an approved return to practice course within the last three years.
- The PREP Continuing Professional Development Standard – nurses must have undertaken and recorded their continuing professional development (CPD) over the three years prior to the renewal of their registration.

Continuing professional development is defined as:

> A process of lifelong learning for all individuals, which meets the needs of patients and delivers health outcomes and health care priorities of the NHS which enables professionals to expand and fulfil their potential.
>
> (HSC, 1999, p. 194)

Although this definition specifically states 'NHS', it is applicable to all areas where nurses are employed.

To satisfy the PREP CPD Standard nurses must produce evidence that they:

- have undertaken at least 35 hours of learning activity relevant to their practice during the three years prior to renewal of registration;
- have maintained a personal professional profile (PPP) of their learning activity;
- have complied with any request from the NMC to audit how these requirements have been met.

> (NMC, 2006a, p. 8)

Activity

Read the NMC publication *The PREP Handbook* (available from **www.nmc-uk.org**), and consider how you might fulfil your PREP CPD requirements when your registration is due.

COMMON REASONS WHY NURSES ARE REMOVED FROM THE REGISTER

Common reasons why nurses are removed from the NMC Register include:

- reckless and wilfully unskilled practice;
- concealing incidents;
- failure to keep essential records;
- falsifying records;
- failure to protect/promote the interest of patients;
- failure to act, knowing that a colleague or subordinate is improperly treating or abusing patients;
- physical or verbal abuse of patients;
- abuse of patients by improperly withholding prescribed drugs or administering unprescribed drugs or an excess of prescribed drugs;
- theft from patients or employers;
- drug-related offences;
- sexual abuse of patients;
- breach of confidentiality.

Activity

Visit the NMC website at **www.nmc-uk.org/aArticle.aspx?ArticleID=193** and find details of recent Fitness for Practice cases that are reported there. Look at the facts of the cases and see how the NMC decided to deal with the allegations.

HEALTH CARE ETHICS (by Ian Donaldson)

The purpose of this section is to outline the theories and principles used in health care ethical debate. However, remember that no amount of reading will equip you with a set of rules to solve all the moral problems you may encounter. Tschudin (2003) believes that ethics can be described only in terms of principles and never in terms of absolutes, while Aristotle is reputed to have said that 'there is a solution to every problem – the only problem is finding it!' It is important to bear this in mind when examining any moral dilemma.

The terms ethics and morals are often used together but, according to Beauchamp and Childress (2001, p. 5), morality refers to 'social conventions about right and wrong human conduct, whereas ethics is a general term referring to both morality and ethical theory'. Both, however, are concerned with evaluating the actions of others.

When observing another person's behaviour and evaluating their actions as right/wrong, good/bad, your evaluation is achieved from a variety of viewpoints. Listed below are some considerations which may help when evaluating actions.

- Legal – actions are right if they comply with the law, wrong if they do not.
- Professional – actions are right if they are supported by codes of professional conduct, protocols and evidence-based practice, and wrong if they do not.
- Religious beliefs – how does God or religious teaching view the action?
- Social convention – does the action conform to customary ways of behaviour in society?
- Practical – an action is right if it is the easiest and most practical way to achieve the desired aim or intention. Conflict will arise if it goes against any of the above or harms the patient.

It is important to recognise that every individual will have differing opinions and views. Burnard and Kendrick (1998) note that the term ethics is notoriously ambiguous, conjuring up different images for different people. However, everyone should be able to express their views, while remembering not to exclude alternative viewpoints. Ethical debate is about individuals reflecting on their own and others' viewpoints with insight and reasoning.

A dilemma is said to occur when an individual recognises that they both ought and ought not to perform a particular action, as there are equally compelling moral reasons for and against that particular course of action. This is made increasingly difficult when individuals have differing views and values, often causing disagreements between those individuals. A good example of this in the UK can be found in the constant debate over abortion – whose rights prevail?

Using theories and principles to guide moral deliberations

There are a wide range of differing moral standpoints but three particular ways of moral reasoning have been extremely influential in the shaping and discussions of health care ethics. These are the theories of Utilitarianism, Deontology and Principles of Healthcare Ethics, the last of which is discussed in the next few pages.

In the late 1970s Beauchamp and Childress wrote a very influential book entitled *Principles of Bio-Medical Ethics*. It is now in its fifth (2001) edition, and many nurses in the UK refer to this text. Beauchamp and Childress suggested that there are four key principles in health care ethics:

- the principle of respect for autonomy;
- the principle of beneficence;
- the principle of non-maleficence;
- the principle of justice.

They argued that by examining a dilemma using these principles the individual will be helped to decide what the right course of action is.

Autonomy

Autonomy, occasionally referred to as self-determination, is defined as 'the capacity to think, decide and act on the basis of such thought and decision ... freely and independently without let or hindrance' (Gillon, 1985, p. 6). Autonomy is seen as being increasingly important within health care.

One reason why respect for autonomy is seen as so fundamentally important is the very close link with consent, both informed and valid legal consent. For example, it is well recognised in the UK that any mentally competent adult has the right in law to consent to any touching of their person (the law relating to children giving consent is different). For an individual to give consent, and so exercise their autonomy, it is clear that information is required to enable an informed decision to be made.

When a person acts to override someone's autonomy, by restricting information or choices, it is described as paternalism. It is always very difficult to know what is the right course of action to take in this type of situation. The principle of respect for autonomy is, however, of central importance when considering a patient's request and must not be treated lightly (refer to the NMC *Code of Conduct* (2004a), which makes very clear the nurse's role in obtaining consent). There are two considerations. First, is the patient mentally competent? Obviously a patient who is not mentally competent may not be able to make an autonomous decision. The implications for decision-making with the elderly and mentally ill patients would be profound. The second consideration rests on whether one of the other principles carries greater weight in that particular situation.

Beneficence

Beneficence is the principle which states that individuals have a moral obligation to act for the benefit of others. This has been the guiding principle for health care for some time, but is utilised to justify acting in the patient's 'best interest'. This causes problems when others make decisions about the patient's or client's care without any reference to the patient or client.

Non-maleficence

The principle of non-maleficence provides more guidance. This principle is 'above all to do no harm'. While, at face value, this seems to be a useful guiding principle, on closer inspection it can be seen that many nursing interventions do cause harm. However, it is clear that to intentionally cause distress is morally wrong and so the principle of non-maleficence is recognised as important.

Justice

The final principle to consider is that of justice. Justice is usually considered in two ways: justice as appropriate punishment for doing wrong (as in criminal justice) and justice as fairness or equality (as in social justice). It is the latter idea of justice which is closest to considerations of resource allocation in health care.

Listed below are a range of different options for the allocation of resources in health care:

- an equal share to everyone;
- random distribution of resources;
- on a first come, first served basis;
- according to need;
- to deserving cases;
- to treat as many as possible.

Some of these options can in themselves create inequalities. For example, to allocate an equal share of a resource to everyone may in some cases be perceived as wrong because some individuals are the disadvantaged as they have a greater need.

Patient confidentiality

A final consideration links back to the issue of patient confidentiality. This important ethical rule is also a major consideration in health care. Breaches of confidentiality should be seen as the exception rather than the rule and occur only after careful consideration. Breaches of confidentiality can be described as either accidental or deliberate. The term accidental implies that the breach has occurred by accident and was unintentional. Deliberate breaches, however, are made after careful consideration of the situation. This consideration must include legal as well as ethical considerations.

A key point stated at the beginning of this section was that theories, rules and principles applied without consideration to the situation will inevitably create unsatisfactory solutions. The key is to look for the fitting answer and this can be done only from a careful examination of the situation.

Activities

1 Consider a situation from your past experience or in your workplace when information was withheld. Was this justified? What legal, professional and ethical implications arose from this type of action? How was the situation resolved? Do you think this was satisfactory – if not, why not?
2 Make a brief comparison of the legal and professional issues that you have had to consider in the past when working as a registered nurse, either in the UK or overseas.

Useful websites

- British Medical Council **www.bma.org.uk**
- Department of Constitutional Affairs (Mental Capacity Act) **www.dca.gov.uk**
- Department of Health **www.dh.gov.uk**
- European Court of Human Rights **www.echr.coe.int**
- General Medical Council **www.gmc-uk.org**
- Health Service Ombudsman **www.ombudsman.org.uk**
- Information Commission **www.dataprotection.gov.uk**
- Law Society for England and Wales (has a useful section on clinical negligence) **www.lawsociety.org.uk**
- Nursing and Midwifery Council **www.nmc-uk.org**
- Royal College of Nursing **www.rcn.org.uk**

Chapter 3

The UK as a Multicultural Society

The aim of this chapter is to explore briefly the concept of culture and raise your awareness regarding the delivery of health care in the UK's multicultural society.

Outcomes

On completion of this chapter you should be able to:

- briefly discuss the concept of culture and associated terminology;

- appraise the customs and factors that may impact upon the provision, delivery and receipt of health care for some service users;

- reflect on the process of communication and how barriers to effective communication may be overcome:

- reflect on your own personal experiences of multicultural dimensions of care;

- outline key issues associated with transcultural care;

- outline current UK legislation important to practice.

INTRODUCTION

The population of the UK at the beginning of the twenty-first century, like that of many European countries, has been shaped considerably by post-war patterns of emigration and immigration. According to the Office of Population Censuses and Surveys (2001) there are approximately 4.5 million people of differing ethnic origin residing in the UK, constituting 7.9 per cent of the population. People from India were identified as the largest of these groups, followed by those from Pakistan, those of mixed ethnic backgrounds, Black Caribbean, Black African and then people from Bangladesh. Given these statistics it is easy to understand why the UK is considered to be a multicultural, multi-ethnic and multifaith society.

CULTURE

According to Giddens (1989, p.31) culture consists of 'the values the members of a given group hold, the norms they follow and the goods they create. Values are viewed as abstract ideals, while norms are definite principles or rules which people are expected to observe' (both of which vary widely from culture to culture).

Culture, in fact, refers to the whole way of life of the members of a society. It includes how they dress, their marriage customs and family life, their patterns of work, religious ceremonies and leisure pursuits. For Berry *et al* (1992, cited Papadopolous *et al*, 1998) culture is the shared way of life of a group of people. It includes those ideas, techniques and habits passed by one generation to another – a social heritage. While Hofstede (1991) suggests there are numerous layers of culture which include:

- national;
- regional;
- gender;
- generational;
- professional;
- organisational;
- social class.

Andrews and Boyle (1999) identify a number of defining characteristics of culture.

- *It is learned* from birth through the process of language acquisition and socialisation. From society's point of view, socialisation is the way culture is transmitted and the individual is fitted into the group's organised way of life.
- *It is shared* by all members of the same cultural group: in fact it is the sharing of cultural beliefs and patterns that binds people together under one identity as a group (even though this is not always a conscious process).
- *It is an adaptation* to specific activities related to environmental and technical factors and to the availability of natural resources.

- **It is a dynamic**, ever-changing process. People do not merely receive their culture from others, they also make it and remake it continually in a process of interaction with others.

And finally Geiger and Davidhizar (1995) suggest the following cultural phenomena exist.

- **Communication** – there is no known culture without a grammatically-complex language with different languages having different meanings.
- **Social organisation** – family systems and religious and other organisation groups vary among cultures.
- **Space** – various cultures have different concepts about social/personal space and territory.
- **Time** – each culture has its own conception and orientation of time.
- **Environmental control** – the values, beliefs and concepts of health practices vary widely among cultural groups. (Remember – although it is not always easy to understand the logic of a particular belief or practice that does not mean there isn't one. It need not be logic based on the laws of Western medical science to be valid and practical.)
- **Biological considerations** – constitutional endowment and vulnerability differ among people representing different cultures.

Activity

How would you relate the Geiger and Davidhizar phenomena to your own culture?

BRITISH CULTURE

What follows is a very brief overview of what might be perceived as the 'British culture' at this time. The country's full name is the United Kingdom of Great Britain (that is, England, Scotland and Wales) and Northern Ireland, and it is usually referred to as the UK.

Population

Britain ranks 18th in the world in terms of population size, with the Office for National Statistics (2007) identifying the population of the UK in 2005 as 60.2 million. However, the population is unequally distributed over the four areas. Inhabitants of England make up approximately 84 per cent of the population, Wales approximately 5 per cent, Scotland approximately 8 per cent and Northern Ireland less than 3 per cent.

Language

English is the main language spoken by an estimated 95 per cent of the population.

Government in the UK

The Queen is the official Head of State; however she only rules symbolically and the power, in reality, belongs to Parliament. The UK's Parliament is one of the oldest in the world, having its origins in the mid-thirteenth century. Parliament consists of the House of Commons and the House of Lords. The House of Commons is made up of members who have been elected by an established democratic process and who represent the population at local area level. The House of Lords is the second chamber of the UK Houses of Parliament and its members are not democratically elected but are drawn from various groups including the nobility and government appointees. The role of the Lords is generally recognised as complementary to that of the Commons and it acts as a revising chamber for many of the more important and controversial Bills/Acts.

At the end of the twentieth century, legislation was passed by the UK Parliament to create devolved parliaments or 'assemblies' in Scotland, Northern Ireland and Wales. Devolution involved the transfer of government powers in areas like education and health (but not, for example, defence) to the UK's nations and regions. The scope of those powers differs between each of the assemblies.

As a member state of the European Union, the UK is also bound by the legislation and wider policies of the European Community.

Religion

Although now a multifaith society, the UK is also recognised as one of the most 'secularised' states in the world. Traditionally the UK is a Christian country with the Church of England being the Established Church in England (with the Queen as its Supreme Governor) and Presbyterianism (Church of Scotland) the official faith in Scotland.

Work

Approximately 75 per cent of UK jobs are in the service industries (which include hotels, restaurants, travel, computers and finance). Most people work a five-day week and, under EU legislation, do not have to work more than 48 hours per week if they do not wish to do so. Employers in the UK must give their workers a minimum of four weeks' paid holiday a year, and must pay them no less than the appropriate (to their age) minimum wage. For example, the main rate for an adult over the age of 22 is currently no less than £5.05 per hour.

Children are not legally allowed to work under the age of 13. Also, between the ages of 13 and 16 years, there is a maximum number of hours they are allowed to work.

Family life

Family size on average is smaller than in most European countries (2.4 children). Family life in the UK changed considerably during the twentieth century, the general trend being a reduction in prominence of the nuclear family coupled with a decrease of the extended family. The number of single-parent families is increasing owing mainly to fewer people marrying and more married couples getting divorced. The relatively high cost of living in the UK, combined with rising costs and shortage of accommodation, is resulting in younger people tending to live in the parental home for much longer than their predecessors. There has also been a rise in the number of single people living alone. People are generally marrying at a later age and having children when they are older.

Education

Education is compulsory for all children between the ages of 5 and 16. Most children in the UK are educated in state-funded schools that are financed through the national taxation system. As with health care, there is some variation in provision between England, Wales, Scotland and Northern Ireland.

Food

The staple foods of the UK are meat, fish, potatoes, flour, butter and eggs, and most traditional dishes will be based on these (for example, fish and chips, roast dishes of beef, lamb, chicken and pork). However, over the past decade there has been a significant increase in the diversity of food that is consumed, particularly food that is associated with Mediterranean European, South and East Asian diets, and many more people are now vegetarian. The intake of convenience 'processed' foods has also increased over this time.

Leisure

As with many other countries, people in the UK enjoy a variety of indoor and outdoor activities, mainly during the weekend and at holiday time. These include watching television, socialising with friends both in the home and outside, sports and hobbies, Do It Yourself (DIY), gardening, going to the cinema, eating out, shopping (excluding food) and travel. The national sport of the UK is football but other main sports played include cricket, rugby, tennis, golf and fishing.

Naming convention

The naming convention in most of the UK is for everyone to have a given first name by which they are usually referred to, followed by a surname which is the last name of either one or both parents. The first name usually, but not always, indicates the child's sex.

National costume

Although customs and traditions involve a wide variety of costumes (for example, the Tower of London Beefeaters) England, unlike Scotland and Wales, has no national dress. In Scotland the national dress for men is the kilt, while in Wales, for women, it is a long skirt worn with a petticoat and a distinctive shawl.

Social customs

People from the UK are often believed to be reserved in manners, dress and speech. As you would expect, the numbers of social customs are vast and vary from region to region. Here are a few as a starting point. Many people from the UK:

- place considerable value on punctuality;
- like to maintain eye contact when talking with or to someone;
- are willing to stand in line, form orderly queues and take their turn as appropriate (for example, waiting for a bus, waiting to pay in a shop);
- prefer others to cover their mouth when they are coughing or yawning;
- shake hands when first introduced;
- instead of calling an individual by their first name, use terms of endearment, for example, duck, love, chuck, mate (which of these is used will generally depend upon which part of the UK a person comes from) – this is normally habit, and not done to offend;
- expect women to be treated with equal respect and status in all areas of life;

- accept that it is OK for women to eat alone in restaurants, wander around on their own, drink alcohol both inside and outside the home and to mix freely with other women and men.

www.statistics.gov.uk
www.data-archive.ac.uk
www.wikipedia.org
www.isc.co.uk

Activity

Note down what you perceive as the significant similarities and differences between the culture of your country of origin and the overview of 'British culture' offered above.

Obviously the more contact you have with people in the UK the more you will come to understand their culture and, just as important, the more they will understand yours.

ASSOCIATED CULTURAL TERMINOLOGY

Terminology closely associated with the term culture includes ethnicity, ethnocentricity, ethnocentrism and race.

Ethnicity

There does not appear to be a single, universally accepted concept of ethnicity and this in itself can pose problems for nurses caring for patients/clients from diverse multi-ethnic groups. According to Jones (1994) ethnicity is generally perceived as referring to the cultural practices and attitudes that characterise a given group of people which distinguish it from other groups, ethnic differences being wholly learnt and a result of socialisation and acculturation.

Ethnocentricity

Summer (1906, cited Papadopoulos *et al*, 1998) suggests ethnocentricity is the tendency to use one's own group's standards as *the* standard. That is, there is an assumption that one's own cultural group is superior to that of others. (This is entirely inconsistent with an ability to provide holistic nursing care.)

Race

Fernando (1991, cited Papadopoulos *et al*, 1998) identifies race as being characterised by physical appearance, determined by ancestry and perceived as a permanent genetic state. Although, according to the Runnymeade Trust (2000, cited Royal College of Nursing (RCN), 2006), the term 'race' is no longer widely used in the human and health sciences in the UK. It is now widely acknowledged as a social/political construct rather than a biological or genetic fact.

CULTURE IN PRACTICE

However culture and associated terms are defined, it is important to remember that culture has historic, present and future dimensions and has immense implications for the care you will provide while working in the UK.

Given the population profile of the UK, you will inevitably find yourself in a position of caring for patients/clients from a variety of cultural/ethnic backgrounds and this will require you to have an understanding of the knowledge and skills required for effective transcultural nursing.

Activity

What is your understanding of the term 'transcultural nursing'?

Leininger and McFarland (2002) suggest that transcultural nursing is theory and practice which focuses specifically on comparing the care for people with differences and similarities in beliefs, values and cultures in order to provide meaningful and beneficial health care. Wagner (2002) suggests that to achieve this requires both health care practitioners and the institution to consider how their practice can guarantee 'recognition, respect and nurturing' of the individual patient's cultural identity. Gerrish *et al* (1996, cited RCN, 2006) suggest this can involve the need to:

- reflect honestly on your own ethnicity;
- interrogate (both intellectually and emotionally) your response to the reality of ethnicity among your patient/client group;
- make explicit any implicit attitudes which might impact negatively on the care given to people of different ethnic backgrounds.

They also suggest nursing professionals need to acquire and develop transcultural 'communicative competence'. Again, at the heart of this lies the capacity for 'adaptability in the sense that the practitioner is able to suspend or modify their own cultural expectations and accommodate new cultural demands...'. This requires the nurse to learn and understand the cultural values, behavioural patterns and interaction in specific cultures.

It is also worth remembering that the NMC *Code of Professional Conduct* (2004a, p. 5) states:

> You are personally accountable for ensuring that you promote and protect the interests and dignity of patients and clients, irrespective of gender, age, race, ability, sexuality, economic status, lifestyle, political, culture or religious beliefs.

This means that every practitioner should seek to ensure that they provide and deliver care that meets the religious, dietary and linguistic requirements of patients while ensuring that the principle of individualised care is not compromised.

The following brief notes seek to either remind you, or raise your awareness with regard to some differing cultural/spiritual beliefs you may encounter in the UK.

Christianity

Christians believe in the Holy Trinity of one God, the father of mankind who created heaven and earth, and who sent his son Jesus Christ to save mankind, and then sent the Holy Spirit to continue his work in human affairs. Christians believe that everything is created and given life by God the Father. Christianity stresses the importance of living a good life in response to God's love. It encompasses many groups and sects but the main ones in the UK are the Anglican Church (which includes the Church of England, Church of Wales and Church of Ireland), the Church of Scotland the Roman Catholic Church, the Free or Non-Conformist Churches (for example, the Baptist Church and Methodist Church) and the Greek, Russian and other Eastern Orthodox Churches.

The Christian holy book is the Bible, the interpretation of which can differ between different sects or groups and so has implications for delivery and acceptance of treatment and care. It is therefore very important that you establish from the outset which Christian sect or group an individual belongs to.

Considerations for practice

Diet

Most Christians do not follow religious dietary restrictions, although some Catholics may wish not to eat meat on Fridays, Ash Wednesday (which occurs in February or March) or Good Friday (which occurs in March or April). They should therefore be offered a fish or vegetarian alternative.

Prayers

Some Christians may wish to receive Holy Communion and, possibly, the Anointing of the Sick, which involves being anointed with holy oil. A private and, where possible, quiet area of the care environment should be found if these rituals take place.

Death and dying

Roman Catholics may wish a priest to carry out the sacrament of the 'Last Rites or Extreme Unction' (anointing). If they are able, the individual may also wish to receive Holy Communion and confess their sins to the priest either before receiving Holy Communion or separately. There are no particular rituals associated with last offices.

Jehovah's Witnesses

Jehovah's Witnesses consider their religion to be a restoration of original first-century Christianity. They accept the Bible as inspired by God. They believe in one God, 'Jehovah', and they believe that the commands in the Bible are very important and, therefore, they try to live by them at all times.

Considerations for practice

Jehovah's Witnesses are totally opposed to taking blood or blood products into the body. This means that they will not accept blood transfusions even in life-threatening situations. However, they will accept alternative treatments.

Diet

Anything that contains blood or blood products is unacceptable, as is meat that has come from an animal that has been strangled, shot or not bled properly. If in doubt, Jehovah's Witnesses should be offered a vegetarian diet.

Patient confidentiality

Confidentiality must be maintained at all times and the patient's permission must be sought regarding what information they would like to be passed on to their family.

Death and dying

There are no particular rites and rituals associated with death and dying.

Hinduism

Largely confined to India, Hinduism is an amalgamation of many local faiths and is inextricably linked to culture and social structure. Hindus believe there is one God who can be worshipped and understood in many different forms. There is a belief in reincarnation in which the status and caste (hereditary or marital social class system) of each life is determined by behaviour in the last life.

Hinduism does not have one leader, a unified code of conduct or creed. Because of this diversity it is difficult to generalise about what a specific individual might believe.

Considerations for practice

Physical examination

Generally, Hindu patients will have a strong preference for being treated and cared for by health care staff that are of the same gender. Privacy during any procedure is very important and female patients may be reluctant to remove clothing. They may also wish a family member to act as a chaperone when physical examination and procedures are being carried out. Care must be taken not to remove any jewellery, threads, etc. without the patient's/family permission as they often have a religious significance.

Personal hygiene

Hindus prefer to shower rather than bathe and should always be provided with water for washing when they go to the toilet.

Diet

Most Hindus are vegetarian, refusing to take the lives of animals for food. Devout Hindus would not eat off a plate on which meat has been served so an acceptable alternative (for example, a plastic/paper plate) might need to be found.

Medication

Medication that contains animal products should be avoided.

Family and individual

As Hindus are intimately integrated with their extended family, there may be issues related to decision-making. Often decisions may be taken by a senior member of the family, or a female patient may wish her husband to consent to any treatment on her behalf.

Hindu patients tend to be visited frequently by their extended family, which can cause some difficulties with regard to the preset visiting times and 'numbers of visitors' policies that exist in most UK hospitals. The family may also wish to perform religious ceremonies with the patient. Privacy should be afforded to allow this to occur.

Prayer and ritual observance

Devout Hindus pray three times a day (at sunrise, noon and sunset). They should be assisted to wash prior to prayers if they are unable to do so independently. Where possible a quiet area should be provided and they should not be disturbed during prayer. Patients may wish to have statues or pictures of Gods at their bedside and these items need to be treated with great care and respect.

Death and dying

Death in hospital can cause considerable religious distress to a Hindu patient and their family. Many patients will have a strong desire, and should be allowed, to die at home. If in hospital they will need to be surrounded by their family, who may wish to read passages from holy texts, say prayers with and for them, and perform required ceremonies.

After death real distress may be caused if a non-Hindu touches the body without wearing disposable gloves. Unless otherwise advised by the family, close the eyes and straighten the legs. Do not cut the hair, nails or any beards. Hands should be placed on the chest with the palms together and fingers under the chin. Religious objects or jewellery should not be removed. Wrap the body in a plain white sheet.

Judaism

Jews consider themselves a nation as much as a religious community. The religious aspects of Judaism are based the relationship between God and man, and relationships between individual humans based on principles of fairness and equality. Religious observance is a means of publicly display-ing a personal acceptance of a close connection between the individual and God. Orthodox Jews are very devout in their faith and adhere strictly to the ancient Torah (holy scriptures/laws). Reform or Liberal Jews believe in the Torah but interpret the laws and scriptures in relation to modern-day circumstances.

Considerations for practice

Personal hygiene

Orthodox Jews may wish to wash themselves before and after eating. Running water is required for this so, if the patient is unable to get out of bed, a bowl and jug of water should be offered.

Diet

Only 'Kosher' food is acceptable to many Jewish patients. Milk and meat are not eaten at the same meal. Meat must be killed according to Kosher ritual and is acceptable only from animals which chew the cud and have cloven hooves, or poultry. Pig and rabbit are forbidden. Fish must have fins and scales and therefore shellfish are forbidden. If Kosher meals are not available a vegetarian diet should be offered.

Prayer

Jews usually say prayers three times a day and privacy and peace should be given to allow this to happen. The Sabbath is a Holy Day on which Jews are restricted in what they may do. It begins at sunset on Friday and ends at sunset on Saturday. It is important to establish the patient's principles with regard to the Sabbath as they may significantly impact on the care offered during this time (for example, a patient may not be willing to use a pen to sign their name on forms).

Death and dying

A Jew who is dying may wish to hear or recite special psalms (particularly Psalm 23). After death the body should be touched by care staff as little as possible and disposable gloves should be worn at all times. Contact should be made with either the next of kin or the Rabbi as soon as possible as they will arrange for the preparation of the body. The face should be cov-ered with a clean cloth or sheet, arms should not be crossed but left at the side of the body with palms facing inwards. Any catheters, drains and tubes should be left in place, as should any wound dressings. Open wounds should be covered. If the patient dies at night the light should be left on when there is no one in the room or bed space. Female bodies should be attended to by female care staff and, if at all possible, male bodies by male care staff.

Muslims

Islam means 'submission and peace' and includes acceptance of those articles of faith, commands and ordinances revealed through the Prophet Mohammed. Muslims believe that the whole universe is under the direction of Allah and nothing can happen unless he wills it. Most practising Muslims follow five main duties or Pillars of Islam:

- faith in one God;
- prayer at five set times every day;
- giving a required amount to charity each year;
- fasting during the holy month of Ramadan;
- making a pilgrimage (Hajj) once in their lives to Mecca if they can.

Considerations for practice

Physical examination and procedures

Physical examination and procedures should generally be carried out by a member of the health care team who is of the same gender as the patient. Privacy during any procedure is very important and female patients may be reluctant to remove clothing. They may also wish a family member to act as a chaperone when physical examination and procedures are being carried out. Consideration should be given to ensure that the patient remains covered appropriately throughout the examination and any other procedure that may need to be performed as part of the care provided. Care must be taken not to remove any jewellery, without the patient's/family permission as it often has a special or religious significance to the patient.

Personal hygiene

In general Muslims prefer to wash in running water so a shower is preferable to a bath where possible.

Diet

Meat must be slaughtered according to the 'Halal' ritual in which the meat is drained of blood. Halal beef, lamb and chicken are eaten but pork, carrion and blood are forbidden. Fish and eggs are allowed but must not be cooked where pork and other non-Halal meat is cooked (for example, in a hospital or care home kitchen). During the month of Ramadan a Muslim should fast between sunrise and sunset. Although Muslims who are temporarily ill or who have a chronic condition may be permitted not to fast, it is important for health care staff to understand that the fasting may still compromise medical diets, tests, etc. If Halal food is not available the family should be allowed to bring food in for the patient, or a strict vegetarian diet should be offered.

Medication

Islam prohibits the consumption of alcohol therefore the patient may refuse medication that contains alcohol.

Prayer

Devout Muslims will pray up to five times a day. Privacy and peace should be given to allow them to do this. Before prayer a ritual wash in running water is undertaken in which face, hands and arms are washed in a predetermined way. If the patient is confined to bed they may need help with their preparation for prayer and a jug of water and a bowl would ensure a source of running water is available. Clothes should also be changed if they have become soiled. There is a special format for prayer that uses a set of hand gestures instead of whole-body movements that can be carried out when the patient is confined to bed.

Family and individual

Muslim patients tend to be visited frequently by their extended family, which can cause some difficulties with regard to the preset visiting times and 'numbers of visitors' policies which exist in most UK hospitals. Many of the visitors may also wish to be involved in the care of the patient, so they should be advised on how they may contribute. As Muslims do not generally encourage men and women to mix freely in public, Muslim patients should not be placed in mixed wards.

Death and dying

As the person approaches death they will expect to have their family and friends around them, which sometimes can be a considerable number of people visiting at any one time. If this happens, caring for the patient in a side room may be preferable. If members of the family are not in attendance when death occurs, health care staff should wear disposable gloves so that they do not directly touch the body. The person's head should be turned towards Mecca (usually south east in the UK), the arms and legs straightened, eyes and mouth closed and the body covered entirely with a clean white sheet. Female bodies should be attended to by female care staff and, if at all possible, male bodies by male care staff. The remaining preparation of the body will be carried out by a member of the family, who should be contacted immediately.

Sikhs

Sikh translates roughly as 'student or disciple' and Sikhism originated as a reformist movement of Hinduism, its founder Guru Nanak attempting to combine the best features of Hinduism and Islam. Sikhs believe in one God and must live a spiritual life and develop their own individual relationship with God by dedicating their lives to doing good. Thus, while on this earth, they should be truthful, gentle, kind and generous, and work towards the common good. They perceive all people as equal.

Sikhs have five 'signs' which they should wear at all times, known as the '5 Ks'. They are:

- Kesh – uncut beard and hair;
- Kangha – wooden comb;
- Kara – steel bracelet worn on the right wrist;
- Kirpan – sharp knife with a double-edged blade (often now in the UK in the form of a badge/brooch);
- Kaccha – long underpants/trousers.

Considerations for practice

Physical examination

Generally Sikh men and women would prefer to be examined by a member of the health care staff of the same gender as themselves, and would wish to remain as covered as possible through an examination or procedure. Removal of any of the 5 Ks must be strictly with the agreement/permission of the patient or their family. When removed treat with great care.

Personal hygiene

Sikhs prefer to use running water for washing and thus prefer to shower rather than bathe. If a patient is unable to use a shower, a bowl and a jug of water is an acceptable alternative. Male Sikhs may also need help to remove their turban (which has to be done at least once a day). Both men and women may need help with the required regular washing, drying and combing of their hair.

Diet

Meat that has been prepared in a ritualistic way for another religion should not be given to a Sikh. Although there are no specific rules about not eating meat many Sikhs are vegetarian and this includes not eating fish or eggs.

Prayer

Sikhs spend a lot of time in meditative contemplation of God. Before prayers the person will want to wash themselves and dress in clean clothes if necessary. A patient may need help to ensure this happens.

Family and individual

Visiting the sick is a duty of the Sikh community so the patient may receive many visitors. Families and friends will also expect to be involved in discussions about treatment and the provision of health care. A patient may refuse treatment or care if the family does not agree with it. Men or women should not be placed in mixed wards.

Death and dying

If a member of the family is not available health care staff should wear disposable gloves to avoid direct contact with the patient after death. Do not undress, wash the body or remove any of the 5 Ks as that is something the family would wish to carry out themselves. Drains and other tubes can be removed. The body should then be wrapped in a clean white cloth/sheet ready for the family to care for.

Buddhism

Buddhism is a way of life rather than an organised religion. Its focus is on personal spiritual development and the attainment of a deeper insight into the true nature of life rather than a set of ritualistic practices. It teaches that all life is interconnected and the path to Enlightenment is through the practice and development of morality, meditation and wisdom. The practice of Buddhism is extremely diverse and Buddhists from different regions will have different interpretations of the central ideas.

Considerations for practice

Diet

Most Buddhists are vegetarians.

Medication

Some Buddhists may refuse to accept medication that contains alcohol or animal products. Some may prefer to use strategies such as meditation to relieve pain as an alternative to conventional analgesia.

Death and dying

A Buddhist who knows that they are dying will probably wish to have their family and friends with them to meditate and chant mantras as death approaches. They will need as much peace and quiet as possible to allow this to happen. After death, do not touch or move the body of a Buddhist patient until advice has been sought from an appropriate source (for example, the family, friends or the hospital chaplain).

(Clarke 1993, Weller 1997, Henley and Schott 1999, **www.ethnicity online.net/**)

SUMMARY

Working with cultural diversity requires knowledge and sensitivity. Generally family members would prefer practitioners to ask about their customs and religious requirements rather than just ignoring them. The most important thing to remember is that whatever cultural or religious beliefs a patient may hold, they will still have preferences and needs which are individual and personal to them alone.

Further information on a range of religions and implications for practice in respect of health care can be obtained from the internet. Your starting point could include:

- **www.interfaith.org.uk**
- **www.bbc.co.uk/religion/religions /**
- **www.nursingtimes.net/nursingtimes/pages/nursingwithdignitypart1**

CULTURE AND COMMUNICATION

Communication in health care is an essential part of demonstrating a caring and therapeutic approach. However, as Henley and Schott (1999, p. 250) identify, 'where there are differences in background, culture and experience, smooth communication is more difficult'.

The communication process

As you are probably already aware, although the process appears simple, in essence it is not. Communication is actually a complex process in which many possibilities for error exist. To remind you, according to transmission models of communication (e.g. Shannon and Weaver, 1949) the communication process is made up of five key components – see Figure 1.

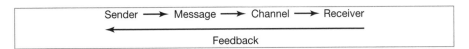

Figure 1 The communication process

The sender (transmitter)

The sender or transmitter is the individual, group or organisation which initiates the communication. All communication begins with the sender, who is initially responsible for the success of the message. The first step for the sender involves the encoding process.

The message

In order to convey meaning the sender must translate information into a message in the form of 'symbols' that represent ideas, concepts, etc. These symbols can take on many forms apart from language/words and include intonations, emphasis, volume, pace and non-verbal gestures (many of which are culturally influenced). It is obviously important for the sender to use symbols that are familiar to and appropriate for the intended receiver.

The channel

The channel is the means by which the sender conveys the message. Channels or types of communication generally come under four main headings:

- verbal;
- non verbal – this can include gesture, posture, gaze, appearance, kinesics, facial expressions, silence;
- tactile;
- written – this can include mass communication through the mass media.

The receiver

After the appropriate channel or channels have been selected, the message enters the decoding stage of the communication process. Decoding is conducted by the receiver. Once the message is received the stimulus is sent to the brain for interpreting in order to assign some type of meaning, or translation of the message to the person's own set of experiences. All interpretations by the receiver are influenced by their experiences, attitudes, knowledge, skills, perceptions and culture.

When the process is followed properly and account taken of any possible cross-cultural styles and processes between the sender and the receiver, it should result in effective communication taking place. However certain barriers that can and do have a negative impact on the process can present themselves at any time during the action. One such barrier is obviously that of language – for example, in the UK where English may be the second language of either the sender or receiver.

Activity

It is beyond the scope of this handbook to provide an in-depth exploration of communication skills and how barriers to communication may be overcome, however the following is offered as a starting-point to remind and inform you regarding these issues.

- Begin and maintain a record of all the unfamiliar jargon (and meaning) that you encounter while in the UK (particularly that relevant to health care) – for example, terms such as 'spend a penny' meaning 'go to the toilet to pass urine'. Add to the record any unfamiliar health care and medical terminology that you encounter and any other issues and factors that you feel may have acted as a barrier to effective communication, and make a note of how you dealt with them.
- Access a copy of *Engaging Ethnic Minority Communities – Communication Guide*, which highlights the languages and potential channels of communication that should be considered with regard to a range of minority communities in the UK including South Asian, Chinese, Black African, Black Caribbean, Kurdish, Turkish and Eastern European. This document can be accessed **www.google.co.uk**
- Consider further reading – for example, **www.En.wikipedia.org/wiki/ Communication** provides a review of factors associated with the communication process (many of which you will probably already be familiar with).

LEGISLATION AND POLICY

In preparation for practice in the UK there are two main pieces of legislation with which you need to be familiar: the Human Rights Act 1998 and the Race Relations (Amendment) Act 2000.

The Human Rights Act 1998

The Human Rights Act 1998 came into force in the UK in October 2000. It represents the translation of the law of the European Convention on Human Rights into British Law. This has meant that, for the first time, the UK has a legislative framework which defines standards for what each person has a right to expect with regard to fundamental human rights and freedoms. The Act covers all infringements of human rights regardless of gender, disability, ethnic identity, sexuality or class and makes it unlawful for public authorities (which include NHS Trusts, Primary Care Trusts, all Health Authorities, private and voluntary sector contractors, social services, general practitioners, dentists, opticians and pharmacists) to act in a way that is incompatible with the Convention Rights unless they are acting under legislation which makes it impossible to act differently. The Convention Rights include:

- *Article 2* – The right to life – The state is required to make adequate provision in their laws for the protection of human life. This means it must take positive steps to protect life in all kinds of situations including admission to hospital and health care. Hospitals are under a duty to take positive steps to safeguard a patient's right to life. Relevant health care staff may therefore need to consider the implications before refusing life-saving treatment to a patient.
- *Article 3* – Freedom from torture and inhuman or degrading treatment or punishment – An absolute right not to be tortured or subjected to treatment or punishment that is inhuman or degrading. How an individual's treatment is classified depends on many different factors including their state of health. Whether or not treatment is considered degrading depends on 'whether a reasonable person of the same age or sex and health as you would have felt degraded' (Department of Constitutional Affairs (DCA), 2006, p. 16).
- *Article 4* – Freedom from slavery and forced or compulsory labour – An absolute right not be treated like a slave or forced to perform certain kinds of labour. This might apply to a situation such as staff from overseas having their passports removed by their employers to prevent them leaving a place of work.

- *Article 5* – Right to liberty, freedom and security of person – Unless a detention is lawful an individual can not be deprived of their liberty for even a short period of time. Detention in this context can include detention in a mental hospital. Acceptable reasons for arrest and detention, in accordance with set procedures set down by law, include: if a person is shown to be of unsound mind, an alcoholic, a drug addict or a vagrant or to prevent an individual spreading infectious disease.
- *Article 6* – Right to a fair trial – Every person has the right to a fair hearing, a public hearing, an independent and impartial tribunal and to a hearing within a reasonable time.
- *Article 7* – Freedom from retrospective criminal law and no punishment without law – Relates to the right normally not to be found guilty of a criminal offence that occurred at a time when the person was not aware that it was a criminal act.
- *Article 8* – Right to respect for private and family life, home and correspondence – Confers the right for each person to live their own life as is reasonable within a democratic society and takes account of the freedoms and rights of others. This right can also include the right to have information about the person, for example official records including medical information, kept private and confidential. This right also places restrictions on the extent to which any public authority can invade an individual's privacy about their body without their permission. It should be noted that this raises issues in such procedures as taking blood samples and the right to refuse treatment.
- *Article 9* – Freedom of thought, conscience and religion – Provides an absolute right for a person to hold the thoughts, positions of conscience or religion of their choice. This includes the right for the person to practise or demonstrate their religion in private or public (as long as it does not interfere with the rights and freedoms of others).
- *Article 10* – Freedom of expression – Expression here includes 'personal views or opinions, speaking aloud, publication of articles or books or leaflets, television or radio broadcasting, producing works of art, communication through the internet, some forms of commercial information' (DCA, 2006, p. 23).
- *Article 11* – Freedom of assembly and association – Every person has the right to 'peacefully' assemble with others.
- *Article 12* – Right to marry – and have a family.
- *Article 14* – Freedom from discrimination – In the context of the Act discrimination is defined as 'treating people in similar situations differently, or those in different situations in the same way, without proper justification' (DCA, 2006, p. 25). Among other issues this includes associated sex and sexual orientation, age, race, colour, language, religion, disability, political or other opinion, national or social origin, association with a national minority, property, birth (for example, whether born inside or outside of marriage) and marital status.

Regardless of status everyone is entitled to equal access to all the rights set out in the Act.

- ***Protocol 1 of Article 2*** – Right to education – No person should be denied the right to the education system and an effective education.

Articles 2, 3, 8, 9 and 14 are particularly important to nursing practice and the NMC *Code of Professional Conduct* (NMC, 2004a).

Activity

Access further information regarding the Human Rights Act 1998 from:

- **www.direct.gov.uk**
- **www.YourRights.org.uk**
- **www.dh.gov.uk**

or through a general search engine such as **www.google.co.uk**. Then consider and note down the implications of Articles 2,3,8,9 and 14 in relation to your practice as qualified practitioner in the UK.

The Race Relations (Amendment) Act 2000

The Race Relations (Amendment) Act 2000 strengthened the 1976 Race Relations Act and includes the requirement that all scheduled public authorities (previously identified on page 65 for the Human Rights Act) must have due regard to the need:

- to eliminate unlawful discrimination;
- to promote equality of opportunity and good relations between persons of different racial backgrounds.

These duties cover all aspects of an organisation's activities, policy and service delivery/provision as well as employment practices. This obviously has considerable implications for working as a nurse in the UK.

Further reading regarding the Race Relations (Amendment) Act 2000 can be obtained from **www.homeoffice.gov.uk**

CULTURE SHOCK

One final thought around culture – given that you have travelled to work in the UK you might find the following of interest. 'Culture shock' describes the impact of moving from a familiar culture to one which is unfamiliar. Some of the elements that contribute to culture shock include changes to climate, food, language, dress, social roles, rules of behaviour and values. The process of culture shock can be identified in five distinct phases. However, individuals may not experience every phase, many 'revisit' a phase and take differing times to make adjustment to the 'new culture' in which they find themselves. The phases are usually identified as follows.

The honeymoon phase

The initial excitement of going abroad continues until some time after the individual arrives in the foreign country. During this stage, expectations for the visit are high and the individual feels stimulated and curious. At this stage they are still protected by the close memory of their own culture.

The distress or crisis phase

The crisis phase may arise immediately on arrival, or be delayed, but generally emerges within a few weeks to a month. It may start with a full-blown crisis or as a series of escalating problems, negative experiences and reactions. Although individual reactions vary, there are typical features. Things start to go wrong, minor issues become major problems and cultural differences become irritating. Individuals can experience increasing disappointments, frustrations, impatience and tension. Life does not make sense and they may feel helpless and confused. A sense of lack of control of their life may lead to depression, isolation, anger or hostility. Excessive emotionality and fatigue may be accompanied by a physical or psychosomatic illness. Individuals find innumerable reasons to dislike and criticise the (foreign) culture. At this stage they may feel they just want to go home and some individuals in fact do. Others cope by using various forms of isolation: for example, living in an ethnic enclave and avoiding substantial learning about the new culture.

The adjustment or re-integration phase

Resolution of culture shock lies in learning how to make an acceptable adaptation to the new culture. An appreciation of the other culture begins to emerge and learning about it becomes more of a fun challenge. Although during the adjustment phase the problems do not necessarily end, the individual begins to develop a more positive attitude towards the challenge. Adjustment however can be slow, often involving recurrent crises and readjustments.

The autonomy phase

Differences and similarities are accepted. The individual may feel more relaxed, confident, more familiar with situations and feel well able to cope with new situations based on their growing experience.

The independence phase

Differences and similarities are valued and important. The individual may feel full of potential and able to trust themselves in all kinds of situations. Most situations become enjoyable and the individual is able to make choices according to their preferences and values (Irwin 2007, **www.ukcosa.org.uk, www.asu.edu**)

Activity

There is a considerable amount of information on the internet regarding the concept of 'culture shock'. You might like to access this information through a general search engine such as **www.google.co.uk** and identify some of the many suggestions offered to help ease the effects of cultural shock. **www.cie.uci. edu/world/shock.html#Tips** is also an excellent site.

Further reading

The RCN provides a very comprehensive resource *Transcultural Health Care Practice* (2006) for nurses and health care practitioners. The document is available from **www.rcn.org.uk/resources/transcultural/index.php**

Chapter 4

Quality Assurance in the UK

This aim of this chapter is to introduce you to the quality assurance framework guiding health care provision in the UK and in particular in England. Quality assurance is obviously expected wherever you work. What tends to be different is both the context and the framework which monitors and guides the assurance around the quality.

Outcomes

On completion of this chapter you should be able to:

- understand some of the main policies and procedures which inform and guide quality assurance in the provision of health care;

- briefly outline the concept of clinical governance;

- understand issues relevant to risk assessment and vulnerable adults;

- discuss the similarities and differences in the processes in ensuring quality assurance in health care in the UK and the country where you were previously working.

DEFINING QUALITY ASSURANCE

According to Marr and Giebing (1994; p. 18), at its simplest, 'quality assurance is about describing, measuring and taking action'. Within the context of health care, Ball (1989, cited Clark and Copcutt, 1997, p. 211) defines quality assurance as 'taking positive action to assess and evaluate performance against agreed and defined standards in order to create and manage a service which regularly achieves desired levels of care and service'. Irwin and Fordham (1995, p. 10) suggest for health care professionals it is 'essentially about practitioners being systematic as well as intuitive in evaluating the care they provide and continually seeking to improve it'.

Quality assurance associated with the provision and delivery of health care in the UK is, in fact, relatively new. Prior to the 1980s quality assurance within the health service tended to be implicit rather than explicit owing largely, according to Dowding and Barr (2002), to the fact that health care was felt to exist for altruistic motives rather than for profit, and these motives were not open to quality scrutiny. International influences in 1984 led to the British government launching the National Quality Campaign for both public and private industries, and the NHS was strongly encouraged to ensure quality control systems were in place. By the 1990s specific requirements and advice on quality were being set out in government health policy. For example, *The Patients Charter* (Department of Health, 1991) set down precise national standards regarding various rights and expectations for all patients. Subsequent policy and legislation, including *A First Class Service: Improving Quality in the New NHS* (Department of Health, 1998a), made more specific plans for progress in improving the health service, especially in terms of effectiveness, efficiency and excellence. These plans reflected the need for clear lines of responsibility and quality management activities incorporating monitoring and continuous improvement. *A First Class Service* also identified clinical effectiveness, evidence-based practice, clinical supervision and continuing professional development activities as specific requirements for health care practitioners in support of quality assurance.

THE ORGANISATION OF QUALITY ASSURANCE IN UK HEALTH CARE

Sale (2005) suggests that within the UK health service there are three main levels at which quality assurance processes take place:

- at national level;
- at Strategic Health Authority/NHS Trust level;
- at the local clinical level.

Quality assurance at national level

Activity

Note down the organisations/agencies at national level that were responsible for ensuring quality of health care provision in the country where you previously worked.

There is no easy way to introduce you to the plethora of organisations and agencies at national level with a mandate to ensure quality of care provision within the UK. However, you need to have a basic understanding/awareness of the key agencies as you will encounter their work either directly or indirectly in your practice.

The Health Care Commission (HCC)

The HCC is an independent body set up by the government to assess, guide and promote the quality of health care and public health (in England) within the NHS and the independent sector. In order to do this the commission is responsible for the following areas.

- Inspecting the quality and value for money of health care and public health by the annual assessment of performance against set criteria in seven categories:
  1 safety (of patients);
  2 clinical cost and effectiveness;
  3 governance;
  4 patient-focused services;
  5 accessibility and responsiveness to care;
  6 the care environment and amenities (well designed and maintained);
  7 public health (improvement, promotion and protection at local level).
  Inspections appraise whether the health care organisation is meeting basic expected levels of performance and demonstrating ongoing improvement.
- Improving health care and public health by:
  - providing information regarding the standards and quality of health care services;
  - investigating patients' complaints that have not been resolved at local level and allegations of serious service failings (particularly where there are concerns for patient safety).
- Informing patients and the public regarding the provision of health care by publishing:
  - an annual rating for each NHS Trust in England;
  - an annual report on the state of health care in England (and Wales).
  (HCC, 2005)

Commission for Patient and Public Involvement in Health (CPPIH)

Sponsored by the government, the CPPIH is an independent, non-departmental public body whose role is to ensure the general public is actively involved in decision-making about health and the provision of health services in England. This is achieved by:

- setting up Patient and Public Involvement Forums (PPIs), of which there are currently in excess of 400 in England (one for each Trust), made up of volunteers from a wide variety of backgrounds and diversity of experiences and skills;
- collecting information from the PPIs and liaising with other national bodies such as the HCC to make recommendations and provide information to the government and public.

www.cppih.org

NHS complaints procedure

The NHS complaints procedure covers complaints made by individuals about any matter connected with the provision of NHS services by NHS organisations or primary care practitioners (GPs, dentists, opticians, and pharmacists). If an individual is dissatisfied with the treatment or service they have received from the NHS they are entitled to make a complaint, have it considered, and receive a response from the NHS organisation or primary care practitioner concerned (except for Foundation Trusts). The complaint must normally be made within six months of the event(s) or within six months of the person becoming aware that they have something to complain about. Foundation Trusts must have in place their own systems for the internal handling of complaints at local resolution level, which may differ from that outlined below. However the independent review stage is still carried out by the HCC.

The first stage of the NHS complaints procedure is known as 'local resolution', with the complaint in the first instance being made to the organisation or primary care practitioner who provided the services. Initially, this may be by voicing concerns to a member of staff or the Patient Advice and Liaison Service (PALS). However, if the individual wishes to make the complaint more formal they can do so either orally or in writing to a complaints manager. A reply from the primary care practitioner involved should be expected within 10 working days, and from a NHS organisation within 25 working days.

If the individual is not satisfied with the outcome they can request and agree on an 'independent review'. In England such reviews are carried out by the HCC. If the individual is still dissatisfied it is possible for the complaint to be considered by a completely independent Health Service Ombudsman (investigator of complaints). Financial compensation, legal action and professional misconduct are not dealt with through this process.

www.adviceguide.org.uk

National Patient Safety Agency (NPSA)

The NPSA is a special health authority set up by the government to improve the safety and quality of care provision. The work of the NPSA includes assessing and reporting on:

- safety aspects of hospital design;
- cleanliness and food;
- safety of the research process.

It also involves:
- supporting local organisations in addressing concerns about the performance of individual doctors or dentists.

In addition, the NPSA has a remit to ensure that 'unsafe' incidents are reported through the promotion of an open and fair culture in the health care working environment, wherever that might be. Where things do go wrong or there are 'near misses' it endeavours to help the NHS learn from the event(s) in order to develop solutions and future preventative strategies. It also is charged with disseminating, at national level, the information gained so that all NHS organisations can learn from this.

www.npsa.nhs.uk

Commission for Social Care Inspection (CSCI)

The remit of the CSCI includes the regulation, review and inspection of all social services in adult and children's services, in the public, private (including care homes with nursing) and voluntary sectors. It also has a remit to provide documentary evidence on the quantity and quality of social care services at both local and national level. Its roles and responsibilities include:

- regular inspection (against statutory regulations and associated minimum standards) of the services identified above plus the inspection of boarding schools, residential special schools and further education colleges (with residential students under 18 years of age) and taking enforcement action when services do not meet minimum standards;
- publication of inspection findings as a publicly available inspection report (accessed through the CSCI website);
- investigating complaints for the areas above;
- publication of the performance ratings of local council social services and judgment on how their services can be improved.

www.csci.org.uk

Activity

Identify any similarities between the information above and the notes you made about your own country in the previous activity.

Quality assurance at the Strategic Health Authority, NHS Trust/PCT level

These organisations are responsible for ensuring that the quality of provision of service is in accordance with requirements set at national level. One mechanism they must have in place through which they can demonstrate this responsibility at this level is a clinical governance framework.

Clinical governance

Clinical governance is a very broad concept. Introduced in 1998, it located quality at the centre of proposed NHS reforms by building on earlier efforts to audit, monitor and improve practice. The Department of Health define it as:

> a framework through which organisations are accountable for continuously improving the quality of their services and safeguarding high standards of care by creating an environment in which excellence in clinical care will flourish.
>
> (Department of Health, 1998a, p. 33)

The RCN identifies clinical governance as 'a framework which helps all clinicians – including nurses – to continuously improve quality and safeguard standards of care' (RCN, 1998 cited RCN, 2003, p. 7). The NMC, in providing guidance on clinical governance, identifies that 'the application of the clinical governance should provide an environment in which clinical excellence can flourish and high standards of care can be promoted'. The NMC goes on to state that 'the principles underpinning self-regulation are inextricably linked to those underpinning clinical governance. Both the professional self-regulation and clinical governance are the business of every registrant' (NMC, 2006b).

Covering the organisations, systems and processes for monitoring and improving services, the key elements of clinical governance include:

- strong leadership and accountability;
- patient, public and carer consultation and involvement;
- clinical effectiveness and a commitment to quality;
- education, training and continuous professional development;

- research and development;
- clinical risk management;
- staff management and performance;
- use of information about patients' experiences, outcomes and processes;
- team working.

All of these key elements are of equal value and importance and all are interrelated.

In essence, clinical governance is perceived as being about ensuring safe, high quality care from those involved in a patient's journey, while ensuring the patient remains the main focus and priority. Baggott (2004) identifies that clinical governance at trust level includes the following processes.

- *Clear lines of responsibility and accountability for clinical areas* NHS Trusts (and PCTs) have a duty of quality whereby the chief executive is responsible for the quality of services provided, and each trust has a named senior officer whose responsibility it is to ensure that arrangements for clinical governance are effective.
- *A comprehensive programme of quality improvement* This includes involvement in clinical audit and confidential enquiries, a commitment to evidence-based practice, and to the implementation of clinical standards in National Service Frameworks (NSF) and National Institute for Clinical Excellence (NICE) recommendations. There is also a responsibility to ensure that workforce planning and continuing professional development is consistent with the need to constantly improve services. Trusts and PCTs are also required to demonstrate that effective communication systems, both internally and externally, and efficient information management processes are in place.
- *Procedures for identifying and remedying poor performance* This includes complaints procedures, incident reporting and clear policies for reporting the concerns of staff.
- *Clear policies for identifying and minimising risk* Trusts and PCTs must have clear policies in place for identifying and minimising risk.

Minimising risk and risk assessment

O'Rourke (2005) suggests that risk assessment in its simplest form is a process which seeks to identify, evaluate and address potential and actual risks.

The increased awareness in recent years that risk assessment and the management of risk within the health and social care sectors in the UK are important factors in providing a high quality service can, according to Milligan (2003), be linked to the professional and government initiative to modernise and monitor health care provision. With a commitment to improve risk assessment a report commissioned by the government in 2000 was published – *An Organization with a Memory: Report of an Expert Group on Learning from Adverse Events in the NHS* (Department of Health, 2000a). The remit of the expert group was to:

- review what was then known regarding the scale and nature of serious failures within health care;
- examine the extent to which the NHS had the capacity to learn from such failures;
- recommend measures that minimised the possibility of failures happening again.

After accepting the recommendations of the report the government published *Building a Safer NHS for Patients: Implementing an Organization with a Memory* (Department of Health, 2001b). This document identified government plans for promoting patient safety and established it as part of their drive for quality within the NHS. Clear links were also made to other government initiatives such as the National Patient Safety Agency.

Further reading on clinical governance can be accessed from the following websites.

- **www.dh.gov.uk/en/Publicationsandstatistics/Lettersandcirculars/ Healthservicecirculars/DH_4004883** This provides succinct but relatively comprehensive coverage of the government's aims and policy principles and implementation of clinical governance in the NHS.
- **www.cgsupport.nhs.uk/** This Clinical Governance Support Team (CGST) website seeks to act as a central resource for all issues relevant to clinical governance.
- **www.rcn.org.uk/publications/pdf/ClinicalGovernance2003.pdf** This RCN guide summarises the key themes of clinical governance and includes case studies to show its application.

Further reading in support of the wider concept and context of risk assessment can also include the following: ▶

- **Health and Safety Executive** The Health and Safety Commission is responsible for health and safety regulation in Great Britain. The Health and Safety Executive and local government are the enforcing authorities who work in support of the Commission. Further information can be obtained from **www.hse.gov.uk**
- **Medicines and Healthcare Products Regulatory Agency** Their role is to 'enhance and safeguard the health of the public by ensuring that medicines and medical devices work, and are acceptably safe'. Further information can be obtained from **www.mhra.gov.uk**

Whistle-blowing case studies available from **www.nhsemployers.org/practice/whistleblowing.cfm** provide a useful opportunity to examine some situations on reporting and addressing concerns relevant to the provision of health care.

Quality assurance at local clinical level

Quality assurance at local level covers a variety of activities including, for example, clinical audit, patients' and users' views and forums and patient advisory services. Further issues such as the Protection of Vulnerable Adults, Integrated Care Pathways and the *Essence of Care* initiative (Department of Health, 2001c) can also be included here.

Clinical audit

The Department of Health in 1989 defined clinical audit as:

> … the systematic and critical analysis of the quality of clinical care, including the procedures used for diagnosis, treatment and care, the associated use of resources and the resulting outcome and quality of life for the patient.
>
> (Department of Health, 1989, p. 39)

In 2002, NICE described it as:

> A quality improvement process that seeks to improve the patient care and outcomes through systematic review of the care against explicit criteria and implementation of change.
>
> **www.nice.org.uk/**

Thus clinical audit is about clinical effectiveness and quality improvement. The key elements of clinical audit are:

- setting standards criteria for a chosen area or topic;
- measuring current practice;
- comparing the results with the standards criteria set;
- changing practice if required;
- re-auditing to ensure quality practice has been maintained or practice has improved.

Put together these elements are usually referred to as the 'audit cycle'.

The fundamental principles associated with clinical audit may be identified as follows. It should:

- be professionally led;
- be viewed as an educational process;
- be a routine part of clinical practice;
- be based on the setting of standards;
- generate results based on the setting of standards;
- generate results that can be used to improve outcome of quality care;
- involve management in both the process and outcome of audit;
- be confidential at the individual patient/clinician level;
- be informed by the views of patients/clients.

(NHS Executive, 1994)

Further information on clinical audit can be obtained from:

- **www.rcn.org.uk/resources/institute/qualityimprovement/ clinicalaudit.php** – for a range of information relevant to clinical audit;
- **www.nice.org.uk/page.aspx?o=233910** – follow pdf link for comprehensive coverage of principles for best practice in clinical audit.

Patients' and users' views

In 2001 the Health and Social Care Act (Department of Health, 2001d) set legislation which placed a duty on the NHS to engage actively with community and service users. The Act established a new framework of patient and public involvement in order to help reduce risk and improve quality within the NHS in England. This included the Patients' Forum and the Patient Advisory Liaison Service.

The Patients' Forum

The Patients' Forum is a network of national and regional organisations concerned with the health care interests of patients and their families and carers. Its remit is to:

- promote discussion about health issues with organisations representing patients and carers;
- improve arrangements for communication, consultation and liaison between health consumers, government and relevant statutory and professional organisations.

Its aim is to:

- provide a means for national and regional organisations representing the interests of people who use health services to share experiences, information and ideas in order to inform and influence decision-making at all levels within the NHS.

It does this by:

- meeting regularly to debate subjects of interest and NHS policies;
- liaising with key players in the health field, including the Department of Health and professional bodies;
- producing policy briefings and updates on issues that impact on patients and carers;
- disseminating information between member organisations.

www.thepatientsforum.org.uk

The Patient Advisory Liaison Service (PALS)

Established in every NHS and Primary Care Trust, this service has been set up to offer confidential support and advice directly to service users, families and carers if they have a perceived cause for complaint or concern. Although not part of the complaints procedure itself, PALS liaise with staff, managers and, where appropriate, other relevant organisations, to negotiate informally and encourage fast solution of the problem or concern. The service is also able to provide:

- information on the NHS and health related matters;
- information on and explanations of the next stages of the complaints procedure;
- a focal point for feedback from patients, families and carers to inform service development;
- where appropriate, referral of patients, families and carers to other local or nationally-based support agencies.

Details of the service are widely available in all NHS areas including GP surgeries, health centres, hospitals, or through NHS Direct.

www.pals.nhs.uk

Protection of vulnerable adults

Risk assessment in health and social care in the UK also involves the protection of vulnerable adults. A vulnerable adult in the UK is defined broadly as:

> a person who is or may be in need of community care services by reason of mental or other disabilities, age or illness; and who is or may be unable to take care of him or herself, or unable to protect him or herself against significant harm or exploitation.
>
> (Department of Health, 2000c, p. 8)

Following a number of high profile serious incidents involving vulnerable adults, the Department of Health (2000c) published *No Secrets: Guidance on Developing and Implementing Multi-Agency Policies and Procedures to Protect Vulnerable Adults from Abuse*. This document provides guidance on actions to be taken within health and social care regarding the appropriate protection and support of vulnerable adults. The aim of the guidance has been to construct a framework in which all relevant agencies are required to work together to ensure strong and coherent policies and procedures are in place, and implemented locally for the protection of vulnerable adults who are at risk of abuse. Abuse in this context is defined by the Department of Health (2000c, p. 9) as 'a violation of an individual's human and civil rights by another person or persons'. The abuse may be a single or repeated act, occur in any relationship and may result in serious harm to, or exploitation of, the person subject to it. The main forms of abuse can be identified as:

- physical abuse (includes misuse of medication and restraint);
- sexual abuse;
- psychological abuse (includes verbal abuse, controlling and withdrawal from services or supportive networks);
- financial/material abuse (includes theft, fraud and misuse or misappropriation of possessions);
- neglect and acts of omission (includes ignoring medical or physical care needs and withholding necessities of life such as medication, adequate nutrition);
- discriminatory abuse (includes racist, sexist, ageist and harassment).

A further form of abuse referring specifically to neglect and poor professional practice is often referred to as institutional abuse. This may be an isolated event of poor or unsatisfactory professional practice through to ongoing ill treatment, or gross misconduct.

The NMC defines abuse within the registrant/client relationship as 'the result of the misuse of power or a betrayal of trust, respect or intimacy between the registrant and the client, which the registrant should know would cause physical or emotional harm to the client' (NMC, 2007, p. 2). Their guidance, which defines the standards of conduct within the registrant/client/patient relationship, identifies zero tolerance of abuse as the only philosophy consistent with protecting the public. It stresses that registrants have a responsibility for ensuring they safeguard the interests of their clients at all times and to protect patients/clients from all forms of abuse. If, in the course of their professional practice, registrants suspect or believe that a client is or has been abused, they must report this as soon as practical to a person of appropriate authority.

Activity

It is recommended that you access and read a copy of the guidelines entitled *Registrant/Client Relationships and Prevention of Abuse* from **www.nmc-org.uk**

The Care Standards Act (Department of Health, 2000d) also outlined a requirement for the introduction of a Protection of Vulnerable Adults (POVA) register. This register was set up in England and Wales in 2004 and is managed by the Department of Health. It contains a list of people deemed unsuitable to work with vulnerable adults. People are referred to and included on the list if they have abused or harmed vulnerable adults in their care or placed them at risk of harm. Any persons placed on the register may not be employed in any capacity to work with vulnerable adults. This scheme currently applies to registered service providers in care homes, domiciliary agencies and adult placement schemes, and all persons working with vulnerable adults in either a paid or a voluntary capacity must be checked against the register. Employment agencies and businesses who supply care workers to these providers are also included. The government's intention is eventually to extend the scheme into the NHS, independent hospitals, clinics and other facilities.

Activity

Further information related to the documents *No Secrets: Guidance on Developing and Implementing Multi-Agency Policies and Procedures to Protect Vulnerable Adults from Abuse* (Department of Health, 2000b) and the protection of vulnerable adults can be accessed from **www.dh.gov.uk** by following the policy guidance/health and social care links or from **www.csci.org.uk**

Having reviewed this document in more depth, take a few minutes to consider and note down what you perceive as your role and responsibilities in the protection of vulnerable adults as a qualified practitioner in the UK.

Integrated Care Pathways (ICPs)

Integrated Care Pathways may also be known as clinical pathways, multidisciplinary pathways of care, care maps, collaborative care pathways or care profiles. They can be defined as 'structured multidisciplinary care plans which detail essential steps in the care of a patient with a specific clinical problem and describe the expected progress of the patient' (Campbell *et al*, 1998, p. 133). The main features of ICPs are that they are multidisciplinary, locally agreed, evidence-based plans (and records) of care which are patient focused and attempt to view the provision of care in terms of the 'patient's journey'. They detail decisions to be made and the care to be provided for a given patient or group for a given condition in a stepwise sequence and within a given timescale. They also incorporate intermediate and long-term outcome criteria and a variance record which allows deviations from the planned care to be documented and analysed. Variations from the pathway may occur as clinical freedom is exercised to meet the needs of the individual patient.

According to Middleton *et al* (2003), initially the development of such pathways concentrated on specific surgical conditions, for example total hip replacement and the more 'predictable' medical conditions such as stroke or acute myocardial infarction, which generally offered a definable sequence of events. Although more and more ICPs are now being utilised for less predictable conditions. Because they are locally agreed and developed it is not possible to provide an overall list of the conditions for which an ICP might have been introduced. However, some examples include:

- care of the elderly: acute admission;
- acute pneumonia;
- inflammatory bowel disease;
- asthma;
- prostatectomy;
- mastectomy;
- aortic valve replacement.

A considerable number of benefits are identified in the literature with regard to the use of ICPs. These include:

- encouraging the translation of national guidelines into local protocols and their subsequent application to clinical practice;

- resulting in more complete and accessible data collection for audit and to encourage changes in practice;
- encouraging multidisciplinary communication, care planning and audit;
- promoting more patient-focused care and improving patient information by letting the patient see what is planned and what progress is expected;
- enabling new staff to learn quickly the key interventions for specific conditions and to appreciate likely variations;
- supporting the introduction of evidence-based practice and use of clinical guidelines;
- providing explicit and well-defined standards for care;
- helping to reduce variations in patient care (by promoting standardisation) and helping to improve clinical outcomes;
- helping improve and even reduce patient documentation by streamlining and combining multidisciplinary documentation;
- disseminating accepted standards of care;
- making explicit the standards of care against which actual care can be judged;
- meaning that full compliance with ICPs meets the NMC standards for clinical record-keeping.

The key steps in developing an ICP include:

- selecting an important area of practice;
- forming a multidisciplinary team;
- comparing current clinical evidence for care of the patient group with established clinical guidelines in all areas of practice;
- developing the ICP (which specifies elements of care detailed in local protocols, the sequence of events and expected patient progress over time)
- piloting the ICP and reviewing the outcomes;
- revising the ICP if necessary;
- implementing the ICP;
- regularly analysing any variants from the ICP (that is, investigating the reasons why practice was different from that recommended in the ICP).

As a nurse in the UK your involvement in ICPs may include:

- using one in practice;
- developing an ICP for a specific condition;
- evaluating an ICP that has already been developed;
- teaching other members of staff regarding their use.

(Middleton *et al*, 2003, Sale, 2000; **www.csp.org.uk**)

> ## Activity
>
> Access further information regarding the development and implementation of ICPs utilising a general search engine such as **www.google.co.uk** You should find the sample documentation available on many of the sites useful for future practice.

THE ESSENCE OF CARE

The Department of Health published *The Essence of Care – Patient Focused Benchmarks for Clinical Governance* in February 2001. Its aim was to provide a tool which would help practitioners take a patient-focused and structured approach to sharing and comparing practice. It was also designed to support measures to improve quality and to contribute to clinical governance within organisations. It focuses on what might be described as the fundamental and essential aspects of care and it seeks to enable health care personnel to work with patients to identify best practice and to develop action plans to improve care.

The tool arose from a commitment in *Making a Difference* (Department of Health, 1999b) to explore the benefits of benchmarking to help improve quality of care. *The NHS Plan* (Department of Health, 2000a) also reinforces the importance of 'getting the basics right' and of improving the patient experience. Initially, patients, carers and professionals worked together to agree and describe good quality care and best practice in eight areas of care:

1 personal and oral hygiene;
2 privacy and dignity;
3 food and nutrition;
4 principles of self-care;
5 safety with clients with mental health needs;
6 record-keeping;
7 pressure ulcers;
8 continence and bladder and bowel care.

A ninth and tenth area that have since been included are:

9 communication (between patients, carers and health care personnel);
10 promoting health.

It should be recognised that all sets of benchmarks are interrelated.

The content of the benchmarking tool

The *Essence of Care* benchmarking toolkit comprises:

- an overall patient-focused outcome that expresses what patients and/or carers want from care in a particular area of practice;
- a number of factors that need to be considered in order to achieve the overall patient-focused outcome.

Each factor consists of:

- a patient-focused benchmark of best practice which is placed at the extreme right of the continuum;
- a continuum between poor and best practice – the benchmark for each factor guides users towards best practice;
- indicators for best practice identified by patients, carers and professionals that support the attainment of best practice.

Using clinical benchmarks

Essence of Care benchmarking is a process of comparing, sharing and developing practice in order to achieve and sustain best practice. Changes and improvements focus on the indicators, since these are the items that patients, carers and professionals believed were important in achieving the benchmarks of best practice. The six stages involved in benchmarking are:

1   agree best practice;
2   assess area against best practice;
3   produce and implement action plan aimed at achieving best practice;
4   review achievement towards best practice;
5   disseminate improvements and or review action plan;
6/1   agree best practice.

The benchmarks are relevant to all health and social care settings. Therefore, the *Essence of Care* is presented in a generic format in order that it can be used in, for example, primary, secondary and tertiary settings and with all patient and/or carer groups, such as in paediatric care, mental health, cancer care, surgery and medicine. It is important that those benchmarking (including patients and carers) agree the indicators that demonstrate best practice within their area of care (Department of Health, April 2003).

Activities

1 It is very important that you understand the *Essence of Care* document as you will no doubt be involved at some point, while practising as a qualified nurse in the UK, in its implementation. The full document can be obtained from **www.dh.gov.uk**

2 Having explored an overview of quality assurance in health care in the UK, make further notes on the similarities and differences between quality assurance processes here and in the health care system in which you have been previously working.

Chapter 5

Evidence-based Practice

The aim of this chapter is to remind you about the importance of respecting and using research and evidence-based practice within your nursing role in the UK.

Outcomes

On completion of this chapter you should be able to:

- review your understanding of evidence-based practice and the need to consider this when carrying out nursing care.

INTRODUCTION

> Most people associate the word research with activities which are substantially removed from day-to-day life and which are pursued by outstandingly gifted persons with an unusual level of commitment.
>
> (Sharp and Howard, 1996, p. 6)

The above is a view, which although stated relatively recently, is rapidly changing. Actually carrying out research may be still the province of comparatively few nurses, but all nurses are touched by the *outcomes* of research projects in the twenty-first century. In past times nursing has relied on a traditional body of knowledge which was passed from generation to generation. However, this rich inheritance has not always been based on knowledge derived from sound research. In some cases practices could have caused harm to patients rather than doing them any good. In undertaking professional roles today nurses need to understand how information derived from research is turned into evidence and thus informs practice.

EVIDENCE-BASED PRACTICE (EBP)

The NMC (2004a) identifies that nurses have a responsibility to deliver care based on current evidence derived from research. The evidence-based practice (EBP) movement started in Canada, primarily in medicine, and has been extended in the UK to various disciplines and professions including education, criminal justice, nursing, social work and social care. Evidence-based practice stems from research, but research is a systematic and rigorous collection and analysis of data to explain a phenomenon, with the aim of contributing to the advancement of knowledge, often in the form of theories (Parahoo, 2006).

The central tenet of EBP is that practitioners combine their clinical or practice expertise and their knowledge of the client or patient with the high quality evidence from research (Sackett *et al*, 1996). It is therefore an opportunity to bridge the gap between research on the one hand, and practice on the other. Figure 1 gives an example of the relationship between the three components of EBP.

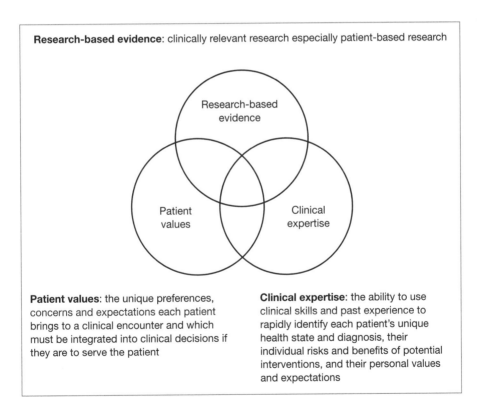

Research-based evidence: clinically relevant research especially patient-based research

Research-based evidence

Patient values

Clinical expertise

Patient values: the unique preferences, concerns and expectations each patient brings to a clinical encounter and which must be integrated into clinical decisions if they are to serve the patient

Clinical expertise: the ability to use clinical skills and past experience to rapidly identify each patient's unique health state and diagnosis, their individual risks and benefits of potential interventions, and their personal values and expectations

Figure 1 The three components of EBP (adapted from Sackett *et al*, 2000; Craig and Smyth, 2003)

Sackett *et al* (1996, p. 72) describe EBP in social care as 'the conscientious, explicit and judicious use of current best evidence in making decisions about the care of individual patients'. They also claim EBP provides 'new types of evidence which, when we know and understand it, creates frequent, major changes in the way we care for our patients' (Sackett *et al*, 1999, p. 6).

Clinical effectiveness

In the UK, the term 'evidence-based practice' is often linked with clinical effectiveness. The reasoning behind this can be seen in the RCN's (1996, p. 31) definition of clinical effectiveness: 'applying the best available knowledge, derived from research, clinical expertise and patient preferences, to achieve optimum processes and outcomes of care for patients' (McClarey and Duff, 1997, p. 31). As you can see this is not dissimilar to a definition of EBP.

McClarey and Duff (1997) believe clinical effectiveness has three distinct parts:

1 obtaining evidence – from research, either published in journals or available on databases; from national level studies based on research, for example, clinical guidelines, systematic reviews or national standards;
2 implementing the evidence – by changing practice to include the research evidence and where possible locally adapting national standards or guidelines;
3 evaluating the impact of the changed practice and readjusting practice as necessary, usually through clinical audit and patient feedback.

Clinical effectiveness is also linked to clinical governance (see pages 75–76). Solomon (2003) states that clinical governance initiatives introduced by the government (Department of Health, 1998a) aim to ensure that care provided is of high quality and has effective outcomes. These outcomes are achieved by employing the principles of EBP. Coyler and Kamath (1999, cited Palfreyman *et al*, 2003, p. 1) add the economic benefits of EBP to their definition as they believe the overall purpose of EBP is to 'provide effective health care within the limited resources available'. The Department of Health (1995, 1997) endorses this by saying that demonstrating clinical and cost effectiveness is a key goal for the NHS, and one means of achieving this is EBP (Palfreyman *et al*, 2003).

EBP IN NURSING

EBP in nursing has its roots in the evidence-based medicine movement but, in nursing definitions of EBP, the patient's views of effectiveness are given prominence. The RCN (1996) emphasises this by saying:

> Evidence-based health care is rooted in the best scientific evidence and takes into account patients' views of effectiveness and clinical expertise in order to promote clinically effective services. This is essential in ensuring that health care practitioners do the things that work and are acceptable to patients and do not do the things which don't work.
>
> (McClarey and Duff, 1997, p. 31)

Such a statement clearly highlights the importance of EBP in nursing. Parahoo (2006) points out that nurses represent the largest group of health care professionals throughout the world and spend considerably more time with patients than any other health professional group. Therefore, as a profession, nursing must build its body of knowledge on solid grounds. Craig and Smyth (2003) have a different view. The huge range of settings and people that nurses work with can be detrimental to implementing EBP; the settings in which nurses work are so varied that research cannot possibly be relevant to all. An example of Craig and Smyth's view is a project where the use of ordinary tap water for wound cleansing was advocated, but the study was carried out in a 'western country' where tap water is 'purified' – the use of tap water in some countries would not be appropriate.

There are many reasons why research in nursing is important. The list below does not begin to cover them all but is a starting-point. EBP:

- establishes justifiable, defensible reasons for nursing actions;
- increases cost-effective practice;
- enhances clinical effectiveness;
- is a basis for assuring quality care delivery (clinical governance);
- improves the patient's experience;
- provides evidence of what does not work;
- provides evidence to support resource allocation;
- supports managing risk;
- encourages academic and professional development.

Offredy (2006) believes that EBP has five stages:

1 a clear question is developed arising from the patient's problem;
2 the question is used to search the literature for evidence relating to the problem;
3 the evidence is appraised critically for its validity and usefulness;
4 the best available current evidence, together with clinical expertise and the patient's perspectives, is used to provide care;
5 the patient outcomes are evaluated.

Again these can be compared with the stages outlined by McClarey and Duff (1997) when talking about clinical effectiveness.

Activity

Where might you obtain information about specific EBP needed to deliver high quality nursing care? Make a list of the resources available to nurses.

EVALUATING RESEARCH

Society's health care needs are constantly changing, which requires that nurses keep their knowledge up to date if they are to provide the best possible care to patients. It is equally the case that nurses need to challenge everyday practices to ensure they are safe for use with patients. A major part of keeping care practice up to date is reviewing or evaluating literature on the subject. Evaluating research always sounds rather daunting for the inexperienced but it can be broken down into a number of simple steps.

Firstly, it is worth reminding yourself why it is important to evaluate research. Perhaps the most important reason is that it enables you to decide the value or worth of a piece of research, given the purposes for which you wish to use it. The following hints for evaluating research articles are taken from **www.rip:org.uk/research_resources/evaluating.asp** This is a comprehensive guide to the process. However, you may not be able to comment on all the questions asked below depending on the focus of the research article, and this is acceptable.

The article

The title

Is it informative, interesting and to the point? Does it address the question that you want answered?

The authors

What do you know about the authors? Do they have a vested interest in the conclusions of the study?

The abstract

Does it summarise the main points of the study adequately and accurately? Be careful as sometimes abstracts promise more than what is actually written in the rest of the paper.

Introduction

Is the problem or purpose of the study clearly stated?

The questions

Are questions stated clearly and concisely? Do they follow logically from the problems? Are they worth answering? Are they answerable?

The literature

Is the background information adequate? Does the author appear to know their subject? Do they appraise related research and authoritative statements? Or have they strung together citations and quotes which support their proposal without consideration of antagonistic arguments? Are specific theories used in order to put the study and potentially the findings into context? Does this theory seem relevant?

Relevance

Is the study placed in the context of current professional knowledge? What is the potential contribution of the study to practice?

Aims

Are the aims stated clearly, concisely and precisely? Are they logically related to the original question(s)? How were they formulated? For example, does evidence from the literature support intuition, instinct and experience? If treatment is being investigated, are the aims related to effi-cacy and safety?

The method

Design

Is the study descriptive or experimental? Is it described adequately? Does the chosen design seem appropriate to you? One or more hypotheses are necessary for an experimental design. Does it/do they follow logically from the original problem and theories?

Assumptions

Are any assumptions being made? Is their use explained? Are they justifi-able and appropriate? Was a pilot study completed? For example, was a questionnaire or special report pre-tested for validity and/or reliability? Were modifications made? What were they and why?

Ethical considerations

Has the author considered the ethics of the proposal? Is the proposed method ethically acceptable? For example, will all service users receive the treatment/intervention they need rather than the treatment needed for the study? Will a control group be required to receive a bogus or dummy treatment of dubious efficacy?

Participants

How were people selected? Are individuals allocated to alternative treat-ment/intervention groups? Is this ethical? Is there an account of how each person was chosen? Were specific criteria used to include people in and/or exclude people from the study? Are they clearly stated? Is the reasoning behind them apparent and sensible?

Samples

Was a specific size of sample chosen (for example, for statistical purposes)? Does it seem adequate to provide sustainable results? If the author aims to make general comments to a population on the basis of the findings, who forms this population? Is the sample representative of this population?

Data collection

Is the method described adequately? Could you replicate it from the descrip-tion? Are the reasons for the choice of method stated? If special report forms, assessment forms, questionnaires, or interview schedules have been used are copies provided with the paper or is an address given for copies?

Analysis

Is the method of analysis understandable? Have statistical tests been used? Are reasons for choice given which explain their appropriateness? Do you understand and accept the explanation?

Results

Are results intelligible enough for you to interpret them and draw your own conclusions? Are they relevant to the stated problem? Does your background knowledge and common sense indicate that they are realistic and feasible? Are 'raw' data given, or only proportions, percentages, etc. after manipulation? Are histograms, pie charts and other graphic representations explained? Are the tables helpful? If results are based on responses to a questionnaire or interview schedule, what is the response rate? Are statistical results included? Are they meaningful? Is the statistical probability of results by chance included? Is it appropriate?

Discussion

Are the results interpreted in relation to the original questions? Are the original questions answered? Have the aims been fulfilled? Does the author discuss any weaknesses in the methodology and factors which may have affected validity or reliability? For example, should selection of sample be discussed? If criteria of inclusion and exclusion need clarification, is the explanation acceptable? Should the advantages and disadvantages of the method of data collection be discussed? Are they? Have you noticed anything that was omitted? Has the author referred to it or ignored it? Have the findings been related to the existing body of knowledge and relevant theory? Are the clinical implications discussed? Was the project funded? By whom? Might the results be biased because of the interests of the financing body?

Conclusions

How do they compare (or contrast) with the conclusions you drew from your interpretation of the results? Do they relate logically to the results?

Recommendations

Are the recommended changes self-evident from the reported results? Could you attempt to implement them, and should you? Is this study an end in itself, or does it suggest further research?

References

Is the length of the list more impressive than its quality? Are any references conspicuous by their absence?

Activity

Go to the Research Mindedness website **http://www.resmind.swa:ac.uk** Click on the section 'Are you research minded?', and undertake the self-evaluation questionnaire.

Now find a research article in any UK nursing journal and review it taking into account the above hints.

FACTORS AFFECTING THE IMPLEMENTATION OF EBP

As indicated throughout this chapter the use of EBP is critical to the qualified nurse within the UK. Indeed the NMC reminds all nurses of this in the final statement of clause 6 of the *Code of Professional Conduct* (2004a, p. 10):

> You have a responsibility to deliver care based on current evidence, best practice and, wherever applicable, validated research when it is available.

However, many difficulties in engaging nurses in research and EBP have been documented (Palfreyman *et al*, 2003). The following have been offered as explanations for this (Gerrish and Lacey, 2006; Craig and Smyth, 2003).

- *Nature of evidence*
  - Lack of clinically relevant research in nursing.
  - What do you do if there is no evidence?
  - Tension between evidence and practice – where research says unequivocally 'X' works, and it doesn't.
  - Research is applied in a set of experimental conditions and cannot be reproduced in real-life settings.

- *How evidence is communicated*
  - Often published in academic journals rather than professional journals which clinical nurses are more likely to read.
  - Limited places at conferences where up-to-date information is presented.
  - Language of research is sometimes a barrier.
  - Researchers fail to draw out the implications of their research for practice.
- *Knowledge and skills of individual nurses*
  - Nurses do not have the knowledge and skills to access and appraise research information.
  - Changing practice is exhausting – how often are nurses asked to do this?
  - Changing practice involves accepting that you may have ceased to be right, maybe for some time.
- *Organisational barriers*
  - Time, heavy clinical workloads.
  - Lack of authority and support to implement findings.
  - Implementing research in one area of practice may disrupt other areas.

Activity

Consider how you would promote the use of EBP in your clinical area. Choose a nursing duty which you have seen carried out *without* regard for current 'evidence', and outline how you would encourage staff to keep updated.

Useful websites

- www.resmind.swa:ac.uk
- www.library.nhs.uk
- www.evidencebasednursing.com
- www.clinicalevidence.com
- www.cochranelibrary.com
- www.rip.org.uk/research_resources/evaluating.asp

Chapter 6

Interprofessional Practice and Changing Roles in UK Nursing

This aim of this chapter is to provide a brief overview regarding interprofessional practice and changes in nurses' roles which have evolved in the UK over the past decade. These topics link closely to other chapters particularly the provision of health care (Chapter 1).

Outcomes

On completion of this chapter you should be able to:

- understand the concept and context of interprofessional practice in the UK;

- appraise the role and function of relevant health and social care professionals;

- reflect on factors relevant to your own interprofessional practice in the UK;

- appreciate why there has been a need for nurses to change their roles;

- understand the main changes that have occurred to nurses' roles in the past decade in the UK.

INTERPROFESSIONAL PRACTICE

The push towards interprofessional collaboration in the field of health care within the UK is relatively new and largely politically driven. As you would expect, since the conception of the NHS in 1948 the provision of health care in the UK has undergone a variety of changes in terms of organisational restructuring, managerial and economic change. Many of these changes have, unfortunately, resulted in fragmentation of health and social care services. This includes both services being managed, at local level, through different governmental channels, each having very different funding arrangements and dissimilar involvement with independent and voluntary sector care. In addition to this professional cultures and forms of accountability within each of the groups have tended to differ significantly.

A perceived solution to this problem, by the government, has been the attempt through legislation and initiatives to develop services at local level that are integrated and require members of different professions and agencies to work together to develop and improve the provision and delivery of health care services within the UK. This principle, despite changes of government, has been central to health and social care provision and delivery policy since the early 1990s. The issues raised in the following commentary will have relevance for wherever you work in the UK.

DEFINITIONS

There are a number of terms associated with or used in the context of interprofessional practice. The following are those you are most likely to come into contact with and the definitions are offered in order to clarify their meaning.

- *Unidisciplinary* – professional groups work independently of one another.
- *Multiprofessional/Multidisciplinary* – primarily unidisciplinary – professional groups tend to function independently of one another, but some discussion and negotiation does on occasion occur in order to solve problems outside the scope of the traditional and established professional disciplines.
- *Intra-professional/Intra-disciplinary* – a professional group that is further divided into smaller sections each with its own area of specialism – for example, nursing adult, paediatric, mental health, health visiting, district nursing. Intersecting lines of communication and collaboration exist between these professional specialisms.
- *Interprofessional/Interdisciplinary* – intersecting lines of communication and collaboration between different professions and agencies (e.g. health and social care, nursing and allied health professionals) are more integrated and all modify their efforts to take account of other team members' contributions.

(Clarke, 1991; Funnell, 1995; Leathard, 2003)

- *Collaborate* – can simply mean 'work jointly on an activity or project' (Pearsall, 2001). Interestingly the term can also mean 'co-operate traitorously with an enemy'.

Activity

Consider each of the definitions above and outline a situation in which you have been involved in previous practice as a qualified practitioner that relates to each definition.

A review of the literature (Leathard, 1994; Soothill *et al*, 1995; Barrett *et al*, 2005), suggests there is a general consensus not only in the political arena but also among health and social care professionals that interprofessional practice can be a positive state and should provide many benefits to both the professionals involved and the clients/patients they care for. The identified benefits of such practice include that it:

- allows for streamlining of services (government driven);
- provides for more effective use of staff;
- offers increased quality overall of service provision;
- provides better use of limited resources.

For the professionals involved, interprofessional practice also:

- provides a more satisfying work environment;
- can encourage development of mutual respect, mutual co-operation and empathy between professionals;
- should improve communication between different professionals;
- allows all members of the team to understand each other's roles and recognise areas of overlap within the traditional disciplines;
- can encourage a greater understanding of the difference between accountability and responsibility of different team members and what is expected of them.

For service users, benefits include:

- continuity of care;
- consistency of care;
- decrease of ambiguity in the information being given to the patient;
- appropriate referral because of the greater understanding of other professionals' roles;
- care being based on a holistic perspective with the best-placed professionals able to meet this agenda.

(Miller *et al*, 2001)

According to Barrett *et al* (2005), if such benefits are to be maximised interprofessional practice will involve complex interactions between the professionals involved and certain factors /processes will need to be in place. These include:

- knowledge of professional roles;
- willing participation;
- confidence;
- open and honest communication;
- trust and mutual respect;
- shared power;
- support and commitment at a senior level.

KNOWLEDGE OF PROFESSIONAL ROLES

In order for effective collaboration to take place, it is considered essential that each team member has an understanding of the role and professional boundaries of other professionals they may be working with. It is likely that you will have a reasonably good knowledge of professionals such as medical practitioners, radiographers and physiotherapists. The following therefore is a brief outline of the role and function of some other professionals with whom you will be likely to work in your role as a qualified nurse in the UK.

District nurse

A district nurse must be qualified and registered in adult nursing and have undertaken a Specialist Practitioner programme (minimum first degree level). These programmes are normally no less than one academic year (32 weeks) full time or part-time equivalent. Community staff nurses can be funded onto a District Nurse Specialist Practitioner Programme via their employing Trust.

District nurses are an integral part of the primary health care team. They provide nursing care to patients during periods of illness/incapacity in non-hospital settings. This is usually in the patient's own home but can also be in residential care homes, health centres or general practitioner surgeries. Patients may be of any age and include those who are housebound, elderly, terminally ill, disabled and those recently discharged from hospital. A district nurse's work is diverse but their main activities include:

- accepting referrals from other professionals and agencies e.g. hospitals, general practitioners;
- assessing, planning and managing the care of patients;
- establishing links with patients' families, carers and, where appropriate, working with them to develop their skills in caring for the patient;
- working both intra and interprofessionally with a range of other professionals and agencies within the NHS, social care, independent and voluntary sector;
- playing a fundamental role in promoting healthy lifestyles and health education/teaching;
- prescribing from an identified list.

www.nhscareers.nhs.uk

www.prospects.ac.uk

Health visitor

A health visitor must be a qualified and registered nurse or midwife who has ideally had at least two years in practice before undertaking the specialist practitioner programme. Most health visitor students are seconded onto a programme by an employer, although a few people may fund themselves.

Health visitors are usually part of the primary health care team and their role involves working with people of all ages in clinics, doctors' surgeries, as well as visiting people in their own homes, especially new mothers and children under the age of five advising on such areas as feeding, safety, physical and emotional development and other aspects of health and childcare.

The main focus of the work of the health visitor is listening to, advising and supporting individuals and groups particularly with regard to health promotion and public health, either of which can involve tackling the impact of social inequality on health, and working closely with at-risk or deprived individuals/groups. Activities will vary according to the nature of the individual role, but may include:

- delivering child health programmes, setting up parenting groups;
- identifying the health needs of neighbourhoods and other groups in the community, such as the homeless;
- working with local communities to help them identify and tackle their own health needs and participate in their own health care planning;
- running groups with a specific health aspect – for example, giving up smoking;
- delivering health improvement programmes which target people with specific needs in such areas as cancer, coronary heart disease, etc.;

- working both intra and interprofessionally with other health and social care professionals, agencies, the independent and voluntary sector (particularly in relation to child protection).

www.nhscareers.nhs.uk

www.prospects.ac.uk

Social worker

A qualified social worker will have undertaken a degree or postgraduate qualification approved by the General Social Care Council. Funding for the student to undertake the education/training may come through employer sponsorship, secondment or from the individual.

Social workers practise in a variety of settings, which includes service user's homes, schools, hospitals and other public sector and voluntary organisations. They work with all age groups and support individuals, families and groups in the community within a framework of relevant legislation and procedures as well as working closely with other organisations including those providing health care. They offer support, advice, counselling and protection to all age groups although they tend to specialise in one specific area. The main areas in which social workers can specialise are:

Working with children and families

This area can include:

- working to protect children believed to be at risk;
- assisting parents who are experiencing difficulties with bringing up their child;
- arranging foster homes or adoption for children who cannot be cared for by their own families;
- helping to keep families together, for example, by giving advice on issues such as drug and alcohol abuse;
- working in children's care homes, and with young offenders in the community.

Working with adults

This area can involve:

- working in a health care setting, assessing the social and emotional needs of patients and their families, helping them adjust to illness;

- evaluating the needs of clients in the community, developing care plans which enable the client to remain living safely and independently at home;
- working with specific groups such as people with HIV or AIDS, the elderly, adults with mental illness, physical disabilities or learning difficulties;
- working to protect vulnerable adults.

Work with offenders

In Northern Ireland, Wales and Scotland, social workers can choose to specialise in working with offenders. Activities again will vary according to the specialist area but can include:

- conducting interviews with service users and their families to assess and review the situation;
- organising and managing packages of support for users of the service;
- recommending and sometimes making decisions about the best course of action for these service users;
- working interprofessionally with health care professionals, other agencies, the independent and voluntary sectors;
- giving evidence in court.

www.gscc.org.uk

www.learndirect-advice.co.uk

Activity

Consider how the roles and function of the health and social care professionals above link to similar roles from your own country of qualification. Note down similarities and differences that might be relevant to your practice within the UK.

INTERPROFESSIONAL SKILLS

Willing participation

According to Hennemann *et al* (1995) and Molyneux (2001) high levels of motivation and willingness of the participants is key to the effectiveness of any interprofessional collaboration. Unfortunately, according to Freeth (2001) if an individual has had an unsatisfactory experience with regard to working interprofessionally their motivation (and willingness) to do so again may be considerably affected, in terms of both engagement and maintenance of collaborative efforts.

Confidence

Writers such as Leathard (2003) suggest that the most basic requirement for interprofessional collaboration must be the individual's own professional competence. They argue that unless professionals feel confident that they are experts in their own field and are so regarded by their peers, they are unlikely to feel sufficiently secure to fully engage in 'sharing' practice with others outside their own professional arena. This obviously has implications for your own practice within the UK.

Open and honest communication

According to Barrett et al (2005) such communication is very much dependent upon internal feelings associated with an individual's level of confidence. Hornby and Atkinson (2000) suggest that the participants also need to set aside any preconceived ideas and judgements they may have about other professions involved in the collaborative practice.

Trust and mutual respect

Stapleton (1998, p. 14) views trust as 'an essential attribute of collaboration', and believes it develops over time through repeated positive interprofessional experiences. The important point here is, therefore, that professionals involved in interprofessional practice might need to allow time for trust to develop. Mutual respect according to Barrett et al (2005), develops when all participants feel valued through explicit acknowledgement of each professions unique contribution to the overall process.

Shared power

Stapleton (1998) identifies shared power as being based on non-hierarchical relationships. However, within the UK, historically, power has tended to be located within the medical profession and although this does seem to be changing slowly, there still appears to be someway to go before they relinquish their traditionally-held power base to a true non-hierarchical relationship with other health/social care professionals (particularly to the so-called 'semi-professionals' such as nurses and social workers).

Support and commitment at a senior level

According to Fieldgrass (1992, cited Barrett et al, 2005) commitment to interprofessional working must also occur at a senior level, as collaborative practice can be expensive in terms of time and resources. If such practice is imposed from a senior level then support for the professionals involved in its development must also come from that level. This, according to Barrett *et al* (2005), needs to involve such strategies as encouraging reflection through clinical supervision, education and training, team development and establishing the guidelines relating to the parameters within which individual professions work.

Activity

Reflect back on your previous experiences of working interprofessionally then, taking each of the above factors in turn, consider the implications for your own practice as a qualified nurse in the UK.

POSTSCRIPT AND A NOTE OF CAUTION

Despite the recognised benefits there are still some difficulties or barriers to effective and widespread interprofessional practice within the UK. These include:

- organisational issues (between health and social services – for example, disparity of boundaries and centres of control);
- operational matters (different budgetary and planning sequences and procedures);
- monetary factors (including different funding structures and sources of financial resources);
- status and validity (social care is directed through democratically elected and appointed agencies, that is, Local Authorities, whereas health care is directed by policy from central government through the NHS);
- professional issues – these are numerous and include:
  - problems associated with differing ideologies, values and language;
  - conflicting views about users;
  - separate training backgrounds;
  - differing organisational boundaries and professional loyalties;
  - inequalities in status and pay;
  - lack of clarity about roles and historical prejudices;
  - professional defence of professions and an unwillingness to dilute them in any way (professional protectionism);
    - differences between specialisms, expertise and skills – this can include medical practitioners.

(Leathard, 2003; Pietroni, 1992)

Ongoing government policy legislation and directives and the inclusion of interprofessional education and training for health and social care professionals seeks to lessen the impact of the above factors.

Further reading

- **www.skillsforhealth.org.uk/viewcomp.php?id=1376** provides further information on competencies for participating effectively in interdisciplinary teams.
- **www.ukipg.org.uk/Educ_Position_Statement.pdf** explores the need for effective regulation of those providing professional services.

CHANGING ROLES IN NURSING

Why the need for change?

The International Council of Nurses (**www.icn.ch/definition.htm**) offers a definition of nursing (see below) which encompasses a vast arena of care that nurses deliver. While it is accepted that not all nurses are involved in all the aspects of nursing described at any one time, registered nurses still need to be flexible, adaptable and innovative in order to be able to respond to the changing needs and perceptions of their patients and clients. In addition, a market-driven health service in the UK and ever-changing reforms require their role to be continuously evolving and changing.

 The ICN Definition of Nursing

Nursing encompasses autonomous and collaborative care of individuals of all ages, families, groups and communities, sick or well and in all settings. Nursing includes the promotion of health, prevention of illness, and the care of ill, disabled and dying people. Advocacy, promotion of a safe environment, research, participation in shaping health policy and in-patient and health systems management, and education are also key nursing roles.

In the UK probably the most profound impact on a nurse's worklife in recent years has been the introduction of *The NHS Plan* (Department of Health, 2000d). This has been the biggest change to health care in England since the NHS was formed in 1948, and it sets out how increased funding and reform aim to redress geographical inequalities, improve service standards, and extend patient choice. It also outlines a new delivery system for the NHS, changes for social services, and changes for NHS staff groups. Indeed one section of the plan actually states it 'encourages nurses and other staff to extend their roles'.

Many of the changes in the NHS today, which include the role of the nurse, have been driven by patients – indeed, they were major contributors to *The NHS Plan*. Patient and client perceptions and expectations of their health care have risen as information on medical and nursing roles have been made more accessible and transparent. However, the changing roles of other health care professionals have also had an impact on the nurses' role, and in some instances has led to the creation of new roles altogether for nurses.

Activity

Revisit the section on *The NHS Plan* in Chapter 1 (page 8) and then view the document *The NHS Plan – an action guide for nurses, midwives and health visitors* (**www.dh.gov.uk**) and review what the government is trying to achieve. Note down how you perceive these reforms might change nurses' roles.

Changing policy, changing practice

The NMC has summarised the changes in the nurse's role over the past decades as follows.

> The practice of nurses, midwives and health visitors is constantly evolving and changing. Nurses, midwives and health visitors have continually adjusted the scope of their practice to meet changing health needs. Changes in health policy, such as the shift towards a primary care led NHS, an increasing emphasis on public health and community based services, together with technological advances and developments in scientific knowledge have required all the health care professions to develop in new ways. These changes have increased the skills and decision-making required of all nurses, midwives and health visitors. What was once unthinkable – nurses carrying out endoscopies, acting as specialists in diverse areas of care such as diabetes and behavioural therapy, working as first assistant to surgeons, and running their own clinics in acute and primary care; midwives developing and leading total programmes of care for pregnant women with severe social and/or emotional difficulties, directing the development of clinical guidelines, and specialising in supporting women and their partners following early pregnancy loss; health visitors co-ordinating community development work, specialising in child protection, and leading multi-agency work on service development for older people – is now

becoming commonplace. *The scope of professional practice* encouraged nurses, midwives and health visitors to take on new roles and activities to adapt to meet changing health care needs. There are few tasks which nurses, midwives and health visitors cannot undertake legally and many former 'extended role' activities e.g. intravenous drug administration, cannulation, venepuncture and ECGs now form the expected skill base of all registered practitioners.

The clinical nurse specialist role in areas such as infection control, tissue viability, stoma care, continence and so on has existed informally since the 1970s. Clinical nurse specialists were seen as experts in a particular area of care or with a particular client group, with post-qualification education and a research base firmly grounded in nursing. The title was not regulated and post-holders usually achieved such jobs through extensive experience and appropriate post-registration courses. Clinical nurse specialists were usually managed within the nursing service. Nurse practitioners developed first in primary care in the late 1980s and offered an alternative service to that provided by general practitioners or filled gaps in service provision such as providing primary care to homeless people. Nurse practitioners diagnose, refer, prescribe and provide complete episodes of care for clients with undifferentiated health problems. In the 1990s, posts emerged in secondary care with the titles of nurse practitioner, advanced practitioner and advanced nurse practitioner. Such posts frequently involve nurses giving care or performing tasks previously done by doctors. For example, in some trusts advanced neo-natal practitioners are replacing junior doctors on the senior house officer rota in special care baby units; surgical nurse practitioners run pre-admission clinics, clerk patients and organise theatre lists, other nurse practitioners work across the primary/secondary care interface and prescribe within protocols for conditions such as hypertension, asthma and so on.

Latterly, consultant nurse, midwife and health visitor posts have been introduced in the NHS. Consultant nurses, midwives and health visitors are expected to be competent to initiate and lead significant practice, education and service development.

Four key areas of responsibility have been defined – expert practice; professional leadership and consultancy; education and development; and practice and service development linked to research and evaluation. Consultant nurses, midwives and health visitors are to have been educated to masters or doctorate level, be registered as a nurse, midwife or health visitor, and hold additional professional qualifications. The development of such posts has been described as a national priority and it has been suggested that these posts should be used to tackle particular service problems and lead service development in government determined priority areas.

In the past, registration was seen as a licence to practise for life. In today's world however the importance of all practitioners ensuring that their skills and expertise remain relevant to the needs of their patients and clients and constantly learning and updating their knowledge and skills is increasingly recognised.

In light of the increasing speed and nature of change in the professional practice of many nurses, midwives and health visitors outlined above, the NMC recognised and responded to the need to consider how its regulatory frameworks protected the public.

(NMC, 2005)

Activity

Having read the NMC statement above list any patient-centred tasks which you, as a nurse, undertook in your previous work that are over and above those you were taught in your initial training. Then list the areas you know where nurses might undertake specialised roles

NEW NURSING ROLES

Part of the reason nurses are changing their roles is that the organisations within health care have also changed their roles, or at least have had to change the way they work, in order to accommodate new technologies, new legislation (both UK and European) and new government initiatives. Some of these new roles nurses are now undertaking are considered below. This is not an exhaustive list, but highlights the concept of nurses working beyond their initial registration.

Nurse consultant and midwife consultant

Nurse consultant and midwife consultant posts were first established in 1999. They are central to the process of health service modernisation, helping to provide patients with services that are fast and convenient. Nurse consultants and midwife consultants are experienced registered nurses and midwives, who will specialise in a particular field of health care. All nurse and midwife consultants spend a minimum of 50 per cent of their time working directly with patients, ensuring that people using the NHS continue to benefit from the very best nursing and midwifery skills.

In addition, the nurse consultants are responsible for developing personal practice, being involved in research and evaluation and contributing to education, training and development. Each consultant role will be very different, depending upon the needs of the employer, but nurses and midwives working at this level are among the highest paid of their professions (**www.nhscareers.nhs.uk**).

Nurse practitioner

The NHS Executive's strategic document *Making a Difference – Strengthening the Nursing, Midwifery and Health Visiting Contribution to Health and Health Care* (Department of Health, 1999b) outlines a new career framework for nurses. This framework includes the development of advanced nursing posts that are intended to extend the career opportunities for expert nurses who wish to remain in clinically focused roles.

Nurse practitioner is one of these posts, and is a nurse who is specially trained (BSc or MSc) to assume an expanded role in providing care under the supervision of a physician. Nurse practitioners work either in primary or in secondary care, and their role is two fold – advanced clinical activities and consultancy. Their clinical role includes:

- direct accessibility to an undifferentiated population of patients;
- using advanced clinical skills to conduct comprehensive physical and psychological assessments of patients;
- making a differential diagnosis;
- initiating and maintaining a continuity of care;
- providing counselling, advice and health promotion;
- prescribing of treatment and medication;
- admission and referral into and discharge from secondary and primary health care systems;
- acting as a resource for other professionals.

(Torn and Nicholl, 1996)

Nurse prescriber

Since 1994 some nurses have been able to prescribe medicines for certain groups of patients. In 1999 the *Review of Prescribing, Supply and Administration* (Department of Health) put forward key principles for the extension of prescribing rights. These principles included the need for appropriate training, regulation and updating, and the need for prescribing to take place within a framework of accountability and competency. From spring 2006, qualified extended formulary nurse prescribers have been able to prescribe any licensed medicine for any medical condition, with the exception of controlled drugs. To be able to prescribe medication in any setting (primary or secondary care) a course of study with assessment is statutory, which leads to an NMC recordable qualification.

Modern matron

(From: *Modern Matrons – Improving the Patient Experience*, Department of Health, 2003)

In 2001, as part of *The NHS Plan*, the NHS re-introduced the role of matron, one which had disappeared in the late 1960s – but this time in a modern, different form. Modern matrons were introduced to provide strong leadership on wards and be highly visible and accessible to patients. They lead by example in driving up standards of clinical care and empower nurses to take on a greater range of clinical tasks to help improve patient care. Also, crucially, they have the power to get the basics right for patients – clean wards, good food, quality care. The new matron role positions nursing at the very heart of the NHS modernisation process. It is part of a profound cultural change which puts the patient first. In such a system, effective front-line leaders are vitally important in achieving delivery.

Their ten key responsibilities are:

1 leading by example;
2 making sure patients get quality care;
3 ensuring staffing is appropriate to patient needs;
4 empowering nurses to take on a wider range of clinical tasks;
5 improving hospital cleanliness;
6 ensuring patients, nutritional needs are met;
7 improving wards for patients;
8 making sure patients are treated with respect;
9 preventing hospital-acquired infection;
10 resolving problems for patients and their relatives by building closer relationships.

THE NHS MODERNISATION AGENCY

Some of the changes were undertaken by the NHS Modernisation Agency, which was established in April 2001 to support the NHS in the task of modernising services and improving experiences and outcomes for patients. The Modernisation Agency was superseded on 1 July 2005 by the NHS Institute for Innovation and Improvement, whose mission is to support the NHS and its workforce in accelerating the delivery of world-class health and health care for patients and the public by encouraging innovation and developing capability at the front line. Detailed below are some of the Modernisation Agency's achievements in terms of Workforce Improvements Themes (**www.wise.nhs.uk**) which might help you appreciate why nurses' roles have changed.

Protocol-based care

The NHS is being transformed to provide a better service to its patients, with a commitment to shaping the service so that it is personalised and puts the patient and the patient's needs at the heart of its re-organisation. Improving the quality of patient care is central to service improvement. Protocol-based care initiatives aim to improve patient experience and invest in the workforce, and provide more opportunities to deliver high standards of care locally by providing patients, carers and health communities with opportunities to become involved in developing services. It also facilitates opportunities for staff to develop their contribution to patient care and supports the implementation of evidence-based treatments.

Hospital at Night

The Hospital at Night model aims to redefine how medical cover is provided in hospitals during the out-of-hours period, with its approach providing the best possible care for patients given the changes in permitted working hours for doctors in training. The model consists of a multidisciplinary night team, which has the competence to cover a wide range of interventions but has the capacity to call in specialist expertise when necessary. This contrasts with the traditional model of junior doctors working in relative isolation and in specialty-based silos. Hospital at Night also advocates:

- supervised multi-specialty handover in the evenings;
- other staff taking on some of the work traditionally done by junior doctors;
- moving a significant proportion of non-urgent work from the night to the evening or daytime;
- reducing the unnecessary duplication of work by better co-ordination and reducing the multiple clerkings and reviews.

Working Time Directive (WTD)

The WTD was a pilot programme set up and funded by the Department of Health in 2002 to test and report on approaches for reducing junior doctors' hours.

Further information about the above, and other work of the Modernisation Agency can be found at **www.wise.nhs.uk**

Activity

Visit the website **www.wise.nhs.uk** and click on the directory of 'themes'. In the full directory click on any subject in the clinical themes which interests you and explore the pages to see how changing roles may impact your personal field of nursing.

ASSISTANT PRACTITIONER

In addition to the enhancement of the role of registered nurses, a new grade of assistant practitioner has been introduced under the Skills for Health Framework, this role being relevant to all health and social care professions. Skills for Health was established in April 2002 and is part of the NHS covering whole health sector – NHS, independent and voluntary employers. The assistant practitioner role involves delivering protocol-based clinical care that was previously in the remit of registered professionals, under the direction and supervision of a state-registered practitioner. One of the remits Skills for Health was given is to develop a career framework for all personnel working within health care. As you can see from the list below the assistant practitioner is at Level 4. What level do you think you are working at?

Key elements of the career framework

- *More Senior Staff – Level 9* Staff with the ultimate responsibility for clinical caseload decision-making and full on-call accountability.
- *Consultant Practitioners – Level 8* Staff working at a very high level of clinical expertise and/or with responsibility for planning of services.
- *Advanced Practitioners – Level 7* Experienced clinical professionals who have developed their skills and theoretical knowledge to a very high standard. They are empowered to make high-level clinical decisions and will often have their own caseload. Non-clinical staff at Level 7 will typically be managing a number of service areas.
- *Senior Practitioners/Specialist Practitioners – Level 6* Staff who have a higher degree of autonomy and responsibility than Level 5 'Practitioners' in the clinical environment, or who are managing one or more service areas in the non-clinical environment.
- *Practitioners – Level 5* Most frequently, registered practitioners in their first and second post-registration/professional qualification jobs.
- *Assistant Practitioners/Associate Practitioners – Level 4* Staff probably studying for foundation degree, BTEC higher or HND. Some of their remit will involve them in delivering protocol-based clinical care that

was previously in the remit of registered professionals, under the direction and supervision of a state-registered practitioner.

- ***Senior Healthcare Assistants/Technicians – Level 3*** Staff in a higher level of responsibility than support workers, probably studying for, or have attained NVQ Level 3, or Assessment of Prior Experiential Learning (APEL).
- ***Support Workers – Level 2*** Staff frequently with the job title of 'Healthcare Assistant' or 'Healthcare Technician' – probably studying for or have attained NVQ Level 2.
- ***Initial Entry Level Jobs – Level 1*** Staff such as 'Domestics' or 'Cadets' requiring very little formal education or previous knowledge, skills or experience in delivering, or supporting the delivery of health care.

www.skillsforhealth.org.uk

Chapter 7

Health Promotion

The aim of this chapter is to explore briefly the concept of health promotion and public health in the context of health care in the UK. You may be familiar with some of the work, but the policy in particular may be new to you.

Outcomes

On completion of this chapter you should be able to:

- briefly explain the concept of health;

- identify the various approaches to health promotion;

- appraise the influence of different factors on an individual's health-related behaviour;

- recognise current government strategies with regard to health promotion and public health.

INTRODUCTION

In working to promote health as a qualified practitioner in the UK it is deemed important to have some understanding of how an individual within your care might define and prioritise health. Such knowledge can help you as a practitioner to tailor interventions to the needs of the person, and to enhance the relevance and success of those interventions. The following are some definitions of health offered in the literature.

> A state of complete physical, mental and social well being and not merely the absence of disease and infirmity.
>
> (WHO, 1946/84, cited Naidoo and Wills, 2000, p. 6)

... freedom from medically defined disease and disability.

(Ewles and Simnett, 1992, p. 6)

Health and disease cannot be defined merely in terms of anatomical, physiological or mental attributes. The real measure is the ability of the individual to function in a manner acceptable to himself and to the group of which he/she is part.

(Dubos, 1959, cited Seedhouse, 1986, p. 41)

Health designates the ability to adapt to changing environments, to growing up and to ageing, to healing when damaged, to suffering and to the peaceful expectation of death.

(Illich, 1977, p. 273)

By health I mean the power to live a full, adult, living, breathing life, in close contact with what I love ... I want to be all that I am capable of becoming.

(Mansfield, 1927, cited Stead, 1977, p. 278)

Activity

Take a few minutes to consider how close or otherwise these definitions may be to your own definition of health.

You should not be concerned if your definition of health differs from those above as it is important to remember that there are no right or wrong definitions. The following factors should also be taken into account.

- *Health means different things to different people* – that is, it is individually defined and we all have our own personal list of priorities. This has implications for health promotion inasmuch as health care professionals should work with the patient's/client's priorities and perceptions of health, rather than their own, if they are to maximise effective/positive outcomes.
- *Perceptions of health may be relative* – to age, life situation, life experiences, cultural influences, etc. Our health priorities will be influenced by these factors and will inevitably change through life, thereby re-emphasising the 'individuality' of health perceptions.
- *Health and illness may co-exist* – for some, health is an ideal state to aim at, whereas others emphasise the need for realism/pragmatism.

- *Health can also be linked to a sense of well being* – the feel-good factor.
- *Health care can be viewed holistically* – Aggleton (1990) stresses that health does not exist purely within the individual: there are elements outside the individual which also constitute health. These don't just influence health, they are 'dimensions' of health itself and, therefore, they include not only emotional, psychological, physical, sexual dimensions but also, in a wider context, social, environmental, and spiritual dimensions. Individuals put emphasis on different aspects according to personal priorities.

Activity

Coming to work in the UK will no doubt initially involve significant changes to your life. Within the dimensions of health identified above, what do you perceive as the priorities for your own health during this time?

Understanding the factors that may affect your health or sense of well being may assist in your maintaining a positive health status while working and living in the UK.

Further reading

Further reading around lay concepts of health can be accessed from:

- www.answers.com/topic/lay-concepts-of-health-and-illness
- www.uta.fi/laitokset/tsph/health/citizens/lay1.html

Both briefly explore some of the theories underpinning lay concepts of health.

HEALTH PROMOTION

In 1989 the Department of Health recommended that health promotion should be a recognised part of health care and that all practitioners (including nurses) should develop skills in, and utilise every opportunity for, health promotion. Subsequent legislation and policy, for example *Saving Lives: Our Healthier Nation* (Department of Health, 1999c) and *Choosing Health: Making Healthy Choices Easier* (Department of Health, 2004a), has reinforced this recommendation. It is now perceived that it is the responsibility of all nurses to incorporate health promotion and health educational activities into their professional roles (Whitehead, 2000).

Although Seedhouse (1997) suggests the area of health promotion is confused, poorly articulated and devoid of a clear philosophy, there are a considerable number of definitions of health promotion to be found in the literature. They include the following.

> Attempts to persuade, cajole or otherwise influence individuals to alter their lifestyle.
>
> (Gott and O'Brien, 1990, p. 30)

> The balanced enhancement of physical, mental, and social facets of positive health, coupled with the prevention of physical, mental and social ill health.
>
> (Downie *et al*, 1998, p. 26)

> Health promotion is about raising the health status of individuals and communities … by promotion in the health context we mean improving health; advancing, supporting, encouraging and placing it higher on personal and public agendas.
>
> (Ewles and Simnett, 1992, p. 19)

> An approach and philosophy of care which reflects awareness of the multiplicity of factors which affect health and which encourages everyone to value independence and individual choice.
>
> (Wilson-Barnett *et al*, 1993, cited Naidoo and Wills, 2000, p. 72)

> Process of enabling people to increase control over and to improve their health.
>
> (WHO, 1986, p. 1)

These definitions overall reflect the current emphasis of health promotion in the UK. That is, it is about a range of activities involving individuals, communities, professionals, government, statutory and voluntary organisations.

APPROACHES TO HEALTH PROMOTION

Naidoo and Wills (2000) identify five different approaches to health promotion within the UK:

1 medical or preventive;
2 behaviour change;
3 educational;
4 empowerment/client centred;
5 social change.

Medical approach

This approach focuses on freedom from medically-defined disease and disability with the use of medical procedures to prevent or improve ill health (prevention and compliance-detection and treatment). It is often identified as having three levels of intervention:

1 *primary prevention* – preventing the onset of disease;
2 *secondary prevention* – preventing progression of disease;
3 *tertiary prevention* – preventing recurrence of illness and reducing effects of illness.

Naidoo and Wills (2000) suggest this approach is popular because:

- it uses scientific methods such as epidemiology;
- in the short term, prevention and early detection of disease is cheaper than treatment (but not always in the long term);
- it is an expert-led, top-down intervention;
- there have been many successes, for example the worldwide eradication of smallpox.

Examples of intervention include: risk education (for example stop smoking) immunisation programmes, screening programmes, rehabilitation and palliative care.

Behaviour change approach

This persuasive approach aims to encourage change in attitudes and behaviour so that people adopt a 'healthier lifestyle' (often as defined by the health promoter) which, in turn, should improve health. This approach puts the responsibility for good health back onto the individual, thereby suggesting that if people do not take responsible action to look after themselves then they are to blame for the consequences. It is similar to the medical approach in that it is an expert-led, top-down approach that, according to Naidoo and Wills (2000, p. 96), 'reinforces the divide between the expert who knows how to improve health and the general public who need education and advice'. Examples of intervention include campaigns to encourage people to stop smoking, eat a healthier diet, improve exercise levels and not drink and drive.

Educational approach

This involves the provision of information and education to enable an individual to make informed decisions. Unlike the behaviour approach its intention is not to persuade or motivate change in a particular direction but, by increasing knowledge, facilitate voluntary choice. Examples of intervention include the provision of leaflets, booklets, etc., group discussions or one-to-one counselling.

Empowerment/client-centred approach

This approach involves addressing only those issues and concerns which are identified by clients themselves and enabling them to gain the skills and confidence to resolve or act upon those concerns. This can involve both self-empowerment and, in a wider context, community empowerment. Unlike the other approaches this is a client-centred approach that is aimed at increasing people's control over their own lives. According to Ewles and Simnett (1999) the process of empowering involves altering how people feel about themselves by improving both their self-awareness and self-esteem. It includes helping them to think critically about their values and beliefs system and it is about having the resources available which enable an individual to make real and free choices.

Scriven and Orme (2001) also note that, in addition to gathering appropriate knowledge and understanding regarding the implications of health actions and having a positive attitude to relevant health-related behaviours, individuals must also believe that they have the ability to carry out these actions. The nurse's role in the process of empowering the individual includes:

- utilising good communication skills (including counselling skills);
- facilitating decision-making through:
  - exploring the client's/patient's existing beliefs, attitudes, values and skills;
  - providing information;
  - negotiating action plans;
- providing ongoing support.

(Scriven and Orme, 2001)

Examples of intervention will depend on the needs relevant to the concerns of the individual/community, but could be as diverse as developing a care plan with a patient to supporting the development of an action group in the community.

Social change approach

This approach involves political and societal action to change the physical, social and economic environment to enable the individual to choose a healthier lifestyle. Examples of intervention include policy, campaigns and legislation.

Further information can be accessed from:

- www.patient.co.uk/showdoc/16 – this offers a range of information on health promotion issues and links to other relevant websites;
- www.healthscotland.com
- www.pubmedcentral.nih.gov/articlerender.fcgi?artid=1117900 and www.healthpromotion.ie – these provide information relevant to their specific areas.

THEORIES AND MODELS USED IN HEALTH PROMOTION

The main focus of health promotion within the UK over the past 20 years has been on modifying those aspects of an individual's behaviour that are known to impact on health. Understanding why people behave in a certain way and how they can be supported to continue chosen positive health behaviours is central to self-empowerment.

There are a number of theories and models that attempt to explain the influence of different factors on an individual's health behaviour and that can be linked to the practice of health promotion in the UK. These include the Stages of Change Model (Prochaska and DiClemente, 1984) and the Health Belief Model (Rosenstock, 1966; Becker, 1974).

STAGES OF CHANGE MODEL (Transtheoretical model)

Originally developed in the late 1970s and early 1980s by Prochaska and DiClemente, this model seeks to identify a cycle or stages of change that an individual may pass through when changing health behaviour. The theory behind this model is that behaviour change does not all happen at one time. Rather, individuals tend to move forward, at their own rate, through a number of stages on their way to successful behaviour change. Each individual needs to decide internally, for themselves, when a stage has been completed and when it is time to move on to the next stage. These stages do not necessarily simply follow each other. Individuals tend to move back and forth between stages and relapse to a prior stage is always possible.

The stages of change

- *Precontemplation* – in this stage, the person may be unaware or barely aware that there is a problem, the cons outweigh the pros and they may be defensive about other people's efforts to effect change in their behaviour.
- *Contemplation* – the person begins to acknowledge that there may be a problem. They are becoming more aware of the personal consequences of their behaviour, are considering change but not quite ready or ambivalent about it, but are more open to receiving information and education.
- *Preparation* – the person has made a commitment to make change, they are beginning to gather information, set goals, and may be developing plans and strategies (for example, buying a book on weight loss or enquiring about 'stop smoking' support groups).
- *Action* – this is the stage where the person has resolved to change and has committed themself to that process by actively taking the steps deemed necessary to effect that change. The amount of time spent in this stage varies (for example, as little as a few hours in the case of giving up smoking or losing weight). The person tends to be more receptive to receiving help and is more likely to seek support from others (a very important element for practice).
- *Maintenance* – the person continues to maintain the change in behaviour and prevent relapse. They remain aware that what they are striving for is personally worthwhile and meaningful, and constantly reformulate the rules of their lives while acquiring new skills to deal with and prevent a return to their previous behaviour.
- *Relapse* – on the way to permanent change of behaviour many people experience relapse. The person may have consciously changed their mind or merely slipped back into old behaviour patterns. Personal feelings of discouragement and failure are often associated with this stage, and can impact significantly upon the person's self-esteem and self-confidence. This needs to be taken into account when encouraging restart of the process at the preparation or action stage.

(Prochaska and DiClemente, 1984; Macqueen *et al*, 1999)

An example of this could be as follows.

- **Pre-contemplation** – the individual has not considered that they are at risk and need to use condoms.
- **Contemplation** – the individual becomes aware of the risk and consequent need to use condoms.
- **Preparation** – the individual begins to think about using condoms in the next six months.
- **Action** – the individual uses condoms consistently (for less than six months).
- **Maintenance** – the individual continues to use condoms consistently.
- **Relapse** – the individual may begin to use condoms less consistently or discontinues use.

THE HEALTH BELIEF MODEL (HBM)

According to Roden (2004) the Health Belief Model (HBM) has been thoroughly evaluated, received empirical support and is considered to be one of the most influential models in health promotion. Initially developed in the 1950s by social psychologists Hochbaum, Rosenstock and Kegals to explain the lack of public participation in health screening and preventive programmes, it was later extended by Becker (1974) and Becker and Maiman (1975) to include all preventive health actions and illness behaviours plus screening behaviours.

The model attempts to explore what makes people take preventive action. It suggests that behaviour, motivation and goal-setting are governed by two key factors:

1 the individual's perception of the *value* of the health goal;
2 *belief* that a specific health action will result in prevention of or relief from illness.

Within these factors there are four specific dimensions:

1 **perceived susceptibility** – the feeling of vulnerability to a given condition (must have an incentive to change);
2 **perceived severity** – feelings about the seriousness of the threat of illness (feeling threatened by current behaviour);
3 **perceived benefits** – belief in the benefits of the action (feel the change would be beneficial and have few adverse effects);
4 **perceived barriers** – balancing the perceived advantages against the disadvantages/obstacles to the proposed action (feel competent to carry out the change).

With this model certain triggers prompt an individual to make a decision to do something positive about their health. The triggers to action can be internal, for example concerns about their own health or a relatives or friend's illness, or external, where they are responding to outside influences, for example media, family, friends or the social environment. The individual then goes through the following thought process:

- they begin by recognising a problem, consider it, relate it to their personal circumstances;
- they weigh up the cost and benefits of doing or not doing something about it;
- they decide on a course of action (making a change or continuing as before) according to their personal beliefs about health – their beliefs about health are influenced by their cultural and social environment and personal experiences which shape their attitude.
   (Becker, 1974; Becker and Haiman, 1975; Naidoo and Wills, 2000)

An example relating to the use of this model could be:

- *perceived susceptibility* – someone close to me dies of lung cancer;
- *perceived severity* – I do get a cough quite often, particularly in the mornings;
- *perceived benefits* – it would save a lot of money if I did give up smoking, relatives and friends would be pleased and my cough should disappear;
- *perceived barriers* – I have been smoking a long time and life is quite stressful, I need a cigarette to help me cope, I know I will find it hard without support;
- *decision* – I will try and give up smoking but must join a group to help me.

Further reading

For further reading on the Health Belief Model and Theory of Reasoned Action, and on other relevant models, access a general search engine such as **www.google.com** and type in each of the models you wish to explore further.

HEALTH PROMOTION POLICY

According to Naidoo and Wills (2000) health promotion has enjoyed varying levels of government support throughout the twentieth century. The extent of this support and its nature have generally varied, as you would expect, according to the political ideology of the government in power.

The most current initiative in England is *Saving Lives: Our Healthier Nation* (Department of Health, 1999c). This White Paper, coupled with *Reducing Health Inequalities: An Action Report* (Department of Health, 1998b), sets out a ten-year strategy for promoting good health and tackling poor health within the UK population. The two overriding aims are to:

1 improve the health of the population as a whole by increasing the length of life and the number of years people spend free from illness;
2 improve the health of the worst off in society and to narrow the health gap between the better and worst off.

(Department of Health, 1999c)

Improving the health of the population

Here the strategy has focused on setting targets aimed at reducing death rates in four main priority areas.

1 **Cancer** – the target is to reduce the death rate from cancer in people under 75 by at least one fifth (approximately 100,000 lives). This is to be achieved by taking action to reduce the main causes of cancer in the UK. Thus action has included promoting a reduction of tobacco smoking and encouraging an increase in the uptake of a diet rich in cereals, fruit and vegetables. Cessation-of-smoking clinics have been established, tobacco advertising has been banned and healthy schools programmes and healthy living centres have been set up to offer support and advice on healthy diets, etc. Early recognition of cancers is promoted through screening programmes such as cervical and breast screening. When cancer has been diagnosed efforts have been made to try and reduce fragmentation regarding the provision and quality of services across the UK. This has included the publication of the National Service Framework for Cancer.
2 **Coronary heart disease and stroke** – the target is to reduce the death rate from coronary heart disease and stroke and related diseases in people under 75 years by at least two fifths (approximately 200,000 lives). This is to be achieved by promoting a reduction in tobacco smoking and alcohol intake, encouraging people to eat a healthier diet, take more exercise and control their body weight. In an effort to reduce variations in health care and improve service provision the National Service Framework for Coronary Heart Disease has set national standards and defined service models for health promotion, disease prevention, diagnosis, treatment, rehabilitation and care across the UK.
3 **Accidents** – the target is to reduce death rates from accidents by at least one fifth (approximately 12,000 lives). This is to be achieved by the introduction of initiatives aimed at making the wider environment safer by, for example, traffic calming measures, speed and traffic management

policies, safer playgrounds, road safety training and compulsory child restraints in cars for children. In the home, people are encouraged to adopt safer behaviour by, for example, ensuring medication is out of the reach of children and promoting the prevention of falls.

4 **Mental health** – the target is to reduce the death rate from suicide and undetermined injury by at least one fifth (approximately 4,000 lives). This is to be achieved by promoting good mental health and reducing risk, mainly by strengthening support systems for those at risk – including the unemployed, young isolated mothers, recently bereaved or divorced. A reduction-in-suicides initiative includes controlling the amount of some drugs that can be bought over the counter (for example, paracetamol), support of those at high risk of suicide and the setting up of specialist mental health help lines through NHS Direct. The National Service Framework for Mental Health sets out national standards and service models and an organisational framework for providing integrated services and commissioning services.

(Department of Health, 1999)

Improving the health of the worst off in society

It is well documented (for example by Black *et al*, 1980; Acheson, 1998) that health inequality in the UK is widespread, with the most disadvantaged within society suffering the most from poor health. It is now acknowledged by the government that, to improve many people's health, there needs to be management and resolution of the underlying causes of ill health such as social and economic deprivation and social exclusion. The government's aim here therefore relates to policies and initiatives to tackle the wider underlying causes of ill health in the UK. This includes a stated intention of reducing poverty levels, improving education and work opportunities and the environment, including the housing stock.

ESSENCE OF CARE

In further support of the move away from treating ill health and towards encouraging the promotion of healthier life choices when providing patient care, the government published a new set of *Essence of Care* Benchmarks in March 2006.

Benchmarks for promoting health

Agreed person outcome Everyone will be supported to make healthier choices for themselves and others.

Factor	Benchmark of best practice
Empowerment and informed choice	Individuals, groups and communities are helped to make positive decisions on personal health and well being.
Education for practitioners	Practitioners have and use their knowledge and skills to promote health.
Assessment of health promotion needs	Individuals, groups and communities are able to identify their health promotion needs.
Opportunities for health promotion	Every appropriate contact is used to enable individuals, groups and communities to find ways to maintain or improve their health and well being.
Engagement	Individuals, groups and communities are actively involved in health promotion planning and actions.
Partnership	Health promotion is undertaken in partnership with others using a variety of expertise and experiences.
Access and accessibility	People have access to health-promoting information, services and/or support which meets their individual needs and circumstances.
Environment	Individuals, groups, communities and agencies influence and create environments which promote people's health and well being.
Outcomes for promoting health	Health promoting activity has a sustainable effect that improves public health.

(Department of Health, 2006b, p. 2)

Further reading

Further information regarding *Essence of Care* can be found on pages 85–87 and more information about these benchmarks from **www.dh.gov.uk/en/Publicationsandstatistics/Publications/Publications PolicyAndGuidance/DH_4005475**

PUBLIC HEALTH

The public health agenda made up the final strand of the government's ten-year health strategy and was clearly linked to the four main priority areas previously outlined (page 126). Public health is concerned with improving the health of the population, rather than treating the diseases of individual patients. The official definition of public health adopted by the government is: 'the science and art of preventing disease, prolonging life, and promoting health through the organised efforts of society' (Acheson, 1988, cited Cowley, 2002, p. 197).

In 2004 the government, following extensive consultation, published its plans on how the public health agenda would progress in England. The Public Health White Paper *Choosing Health: Making Healthy Choices Easier* (Department of Health, 2004a) outlined three key principles that were to underpin the strategy. They were:

1 *informed choice* – including providing credible and trustworthy information to help people to make informed choices;
2 *personalisation* – including support and services to be tailored to meet the realities of people's lives;
3 *working together* – involving partnerships across the NHS, local government, the independent sector, voluntary sector, businesses, local communities, the media, religious groups, etc.

A set of priorities were established that were to be targeted through government, the media and locally-based campaigns, and initiatives and encouragement of individual responsibility in the identified areas. The priorities were identified as:

- reducing the number of people who smoke;
- reducing obesity and improving diet and nutrition;
- increasing exercise;
- encouraging and supporting sensible drinking;
- improving sexual health;
- improving mental health.

Nurses and, in particular, health visitors have an important part to play in the public health agenda. In order to achieve this, the government has sought to modernise the health visitors' role to enable them to build on their work with individuals, families and communities to further improve health and tackle health inequalities.

A considerable number of the strategies and initiatives outlined in both *Saving Lives: Our Healthier Nation* (Department of Health, 1999c) and *Choosing Health: Making Healthy Choices Easier* (Department of Health,

2004c) have now been introduced. How successful they have been is still the subject of ongoing research.

National Institute for Health and Clinical Excellence (NICE)

NICE provides public health guidance for staff working in the NHS, private and voluntary sectors and for Local Authorities. In general, nurses and other health care professionals are expected to follow this guidance, unless the recommendations are not deemed suitable for someone because of their medical condition, general health, wishes or a combination of these. There are two types of NICE public health guidance:

1 *public health intervention guidance* – recommendations on types of activities provided by local organisations that may help reduce people's risk of developing a disease or condition or help maintain a healthy lifestyle;
2 *public health programme guidance* – this covers broader action for the promotion of good health and the prevention of ill health. The guidance may focus on a topic, for example smoking, on a particular population, for example older people, or on a particular setting, for example the workplace.

www.nice.org.uk

Further information

- If you wish to explore issues around public health and policy further a good starting-point for details regarding public health guidance could be: **www.nice.org.uk**
- On the state of public health, the *Annual Report of Chief Medical Officer* (2005) is available from **www.dh.gov.uk/en/publicationsand statistics/Publications/AnnualReports/DH_4137366**
  This is a report that highlights health challenges that face the UK and details the progress made in key action areas.
- *Public Health in England* (2007) is available from **www.dh.gov.uk**
  This provides an overview of current and regional public health, international comparisons and links to further relevant information.
- Information regarding Scotland, Wales and Northern Ireland can be obtained from **www.show.scot.nhs.uk/publicationsindex.htm**, **www.wales.nhs.uk** and **www.dhsspsni.gov.uk** – follow public health links.

Chapter 8

Nurse Education, Mentoring and Preceptorship in the UK

This chapter seeks to provide an overview of the preparation nurses undertake during their pre-registration programmes in the UK. It also provides an insight into the registered nurse's role in supporting these students, and others on post-qualifying courses.

Outcomes

On completion of this chapter you should be able to:

- have an outline view of programmes leading to nurse registration in the UK;

- understand the need for mentorship and preceptorship in nursing;

- define the qualities required to be a good mentor/preceptor.

NURSE EDUCATION IN THE UK

Nurse education in the UK prior to the 1990s was a traditional 'apprentice' style training where nurses were based in a school of nursing within the hospital where they carried out their clinical work. There were then two levels of nurse qualification – registered nurse (first-level nurse) and enrolled nurse (second-level nurse), the former requiring three years of training, and the latter a more practically-based two-year training programme. However, in the 1980s, there was a push towards establishing nursing in a 'more professional light' and a recognition that nurses were taking on work more traditionally carried out by doctors, while health care assistants were undertaking work which had previously been carried out by registered nurses. This was coupled with the appreciation that there were common elements that underpinned all nursing practice whichever 'branch' (mental health, learning disability, adult, child health) of nursing was studied, and that there needed to be an increased focus on essential skills such as communication, reflective practice, research awareness and the use of evidence-based practice (RCN, 2004).

The 1990s saw the advent of Project 2000 – a new style of nurse training which transformed pre-registration nurse education, and continues to do so. Nurses now study in Higher Education Institutes and exit their programme not only with a first-level professional nursing qualification (RN), but with a Higher Education qualification as well. At the same time as Project 2000 commenced, enrolled nurse training ceased and schools of nursing within hospitals were transferred to universities. Subsequently, preparation for midwifery became a 'direct entry' programme, which enables students to undertake three years of training without holding a previous nursing registration.

Currently in the UK programmes of study to prepare nurses for registration are normally completed in three years of full-time study. Programmes are offered at diploma, advanced diploma or degree level, the level the student studies at usually being dependent on their academic qualifications on leaving school. Students have to be $17\frac{1}{2}$ years old when they start a programme, but there is no upper age limit for applicants, and mature students without formal qualifications, or those who have not undertaken academic study in recent years, can apply following successful completion of an Access to Higher Education course at a College of Further Education. Each Higher Education Institution is responsible for its own recruitment and admissions policy, and sets its own entry requirements. The NMC simply stipulates that applicants must provide evidence of literacy and numeracy, which may be integral to academic or vocational qualifications, or may be shown in Key Skills abilities (level 3) (Nursing and Midwifery Admissions Service, 2007). However, the NMC is clear that Higher Education Institutions must satisfy themselves 'that applicants have good health and good character for safe and effective practice' (NMAS, 2007).

Students studying at all academic levels initially complete a common foundation programme within their first year, where aspects of nursing common to all areas of practice are studied. They then specialise for the remaining two years in either adult, child, mental health or learning disabilities nursing. Although students identify on commencement of the programme the branch of nursing in which they wish ultimately to register, there is the facility for them to transfer branches at the end of the first year. Likewise, if a student excels on a diploma or advanced diploma programme they can transfer to a degree programme, or vice versa if the level of study proves too challenging for a student initially enrolled on the degree programme.

Clinical practice placements are an essential and integral part of the programme and learners spend 50 per cent of their time studying theoretical aspects and 50 per cent clinical aspects (**www.practicebasedlearning.org** 2007). Therefore, students experience a range of clinical placements during each year. During their practice hours students are deemed supernumerary and are not included in the number of staff in the clinical placement. They are assessed in practice by their mentor via a set of competencies issued by the NMC (a series of standards that students have to achieve both during and at the end of their three-year programme). The competencies fall into four domains of practice:

1 professional and ethical;
2 care delivery;
3 care management;
4 personal and professional development.

(NMC, 2004c)

Standards of proficiency for nursing

The NMC is responsible for setting standards of proficiency that define the overarching principles of being able to practise as a nurse, and must be achieved before students are eligible to join the register. These are outlined below:

- manage oneself, one's practice, and that of others, in accordance with *The NMC Code of Professional Conduct: Standards for Conduct, Performance and Ethics* (the Code – NMC, 2004a), recognising one's own abilities and limitations;
- practise in accordance with an ethical and legal framework which ensures the primacy of patient and client interest and well being and respects confidentiality;
- practise in a fair and anti-discriminatory way, acknowledging the differences in beliefs and cultural practices of individuals or groups;
- engage in, develop and disengage from therapeutic relationships through the use of appropriate communication and interpersonal skills;
- create and utilise opportunities to promote the health and well being of patients, clients and groups;
- undertake and document a comprehensive, systematic and accurate nursing assessment of the physical, psychological, social and spiritual needs of patients, clients and communities;
- formulate and document a plan of nursing care, where possible in partnership with patients, clients, their carers and family and friends, within a framework of informed consent;

- based on the best available evidence, apply knowledge and an appropriate repertoire of skills indicative of safe nursing practice;
- provide a rationale for the nursing care delivered which takes account of social, cultural, spiritual, legal, political and economic influences;
- evaluate and document the outcomes of nursing and other interventions;
- demonstrate sound clinical judgement across a range of differing professional and care delivery contexts;
- contribute to public protection by creating and maintaining a safe environment of care through the use of quality assurance and risk management strategies;
- demonstrate knowledge of effective interprofessional working practices which respect and utilise the contributions of members of the health and social care team;
- delegate duties to others, as appropriate, ensuring that they are supervised and monitored;
- demonstrate key skills;
- demonstrate a commitment to the need for continuing professional development and personal supervision activities in order to enhance knowledge, skills, values and attitudes needed for safe and effective nursing practice;
- enhance the professional development and safe practice of others through peer support, leadership, supervision and teaching.

(NMC, 2004c, p. 5)

Funding

Unlike the apprenticeship system, where students were salaried, students of today receive grants or bursaries to support them throughout their programme. Those undertaking diploma and advanced diploma courses receive a non-means-tested bursary which is a flat-rate grant with no contribution from the student or their family. Degree-level nursing students, like all degree students, receive support in the form of a means-tested bursary, supplemented by a reduced-rate repayable student loan. Unlike other university programmes, the NHS pays the tuition fees to the university, rather than the individual student.

Further reading

If you wish to know more about pre-registration nursing programmes there is an excellent section on the Practice Based Learning website **www.practicebasedlearning.org** (click on Case Studies, then click on Nursing Case Study), this discusses practice education in nursing and includes topics such as the pre-registration nursing courses in the UK and mentorship. Alternatively visit the NMC website – **www.nmc-uk.org**

MENTORSHIP

The role of the mentor/preceptor

Many practice-based professions, including nursing, traditionally rely on clinical staff to support, supervise and teach students in practice settings – the underlying rationale being that in working alongside practitioners, students will learn from experts in a safe, supportive and educationally adjusted environment (Benner, 1984).

The form of support afforded to students can be difficult to define by name, and many different terms are used in different countries – mentor, practice educator, supervisor, assessor, facilitator, preceptor, to name a few. In the UK, within nursing, the term mentor is generally used to describe a person who supports and assesses student nurses, while the term preceptor is used for a supporter of a post-registration nurse during their first few months after qualifying.

The most popular definition of a mentor comes from the document *Preparation for Mentors and Teachers* (ENB/Department of Health, 2001, p. 6), which states 'a mentor is a nurse who facilitates learning and supervises and assesses students in the practice setting'. The NMC states that all students on pre-registration nursing education programmes *must* be supported and assessed by qualified mentors (NMC, 2006b). The mentor must have the equivalent of one year's full-time post-registration experience, be on the same part of the register as their student, and have undertaken specific preparation for the role comprising a mentorship course accredited by a Higher Education Institution. The content of such a mentorship course must include:

- establishing effective working relationships;
- facilitation of learning;
- assessment and accountability;
- evaluation of learning;
- creating an environment for learning;
- context of practice;
- evidence-based practice;
- leadership.

(NMC, 2006b, p. 6)

In August 2006 the NMC document: *Standards to Support Learning and Assessment in Practice* (NMC, 2006b), reiterated the need for all students to have mentors, but also introduced the new role of a 'sign-off' mentor. The sign-off mentor, who has undergone a mentor preparation course and meets additional specific criteria, is responsible (and accountable) for 'signing-off' a student at the end of their training period and confirming they have achieved all their competencies for entry to the register. However, despite the NMC's ruling, there is an expectation and requirement that all registered nurses play a key part in the preparation of students for registration within the profession. This is emphasised in *The Code of Professional Conduct* (clause 6.4):

> You have a responsibility to facilitate students of nursing, midwifery and specialist community public health nursing and others to develop their competence.
>
> (NMC, 2004a, p. 10)

Activity

Many of you may have already undertaken a role similar to that of a mentor, so take time to complete the following activity.

- List any qualities you can think of which are desirable in a mentor.
- Can you think of any obstacles to effective mentoring?
- What are the benefits to the student?
- What are the benefits for the mentor?

If you wish to know more about mentoring visit the Practice Based Learning website at **www.practicebasedlearning.org**. Click on resources, then learning materials, then mentoring.

PRECEPTORSHIP

There is a general acknowledgement that all professions need a period of preceptorship following qualification for professional registration, and this of course includes nursing. The UKCC (now NMC) report *Fitness for Practice*, published in 1999, highlighted this in saying: 'All newly-qualified registrants should receive a properly supported period of induction and preceptorship when they begin their employment' (UKCC, 1999, p. 1). The UKCC further added that the health care professions should actively be encouraged to learn with and from one another, which is reflected in the increasing number of preceptorship programmes available.

Preceptorship comes under the banner of 'lifelong learning' and the NMC has republished their document *Supporting Nurses and Midwives through Lifelong Learning* (NMC, 2005b). According to this document the NMC believes that all newly registered nurses and midwives should have a formal period of support, under the guidance of a preceptor. The precise length of time will vary according to individual need and local circumstances, but the NMC (2005b) believes that four months is a suitable time. In many ways, every time a newly qualified nurse works alongside more experienced professional colleagues, they can learn from their colleagues and be guided by them as the newly qualified nurse further develops their own skills and confidence.

Formal preceptorship, however, means that the newly registered nurse is allocated a named individual, working in the same area of practice, who is on hand to guide, help, advise and support. The NMC states (2005b, p. 1) that: 'this doesn't mean that they accompany the newly registered nurse everywhere they go and constantly look over their shoulder, but it does mean they can be called if help is needed with a procedure or a situation not encountered before; or if they simply feel that they need support and guidance'.

Preceptors, like mentors, should be first-level registered nurses who have had at least twelve months' experience as a registered nurse and understand the concept of preceptorship. There are no formal qualifications to be a preceptor, but preceptors must:

- know about the newly registered nurse's training and experience and be able to identify learning needs;
- help the newly registered nurse apply knowledge to practice;
- be able to act as a resource to facilitate the newly qualified nurse's professional development.

(NMC, 2006c, p. 1)

Preceptorship is not a mandatory requirement and the NMC has no power to enforce the system, but most NHS Trusts run preceptorship courses within their organisations. Some courses are affiliated to universities and nurses can gain academic credit for successfully completing the scheme of study. It is envisaged that all newly qualified staff complete any preceptorship course within one year of qualifying, and that the majority of content will be practice based.

Activity

Think back to when you first qualified. What were the major aspects of your role that caused you concern? Did you have a preceptorship (or similar) course?

Useful websites

- www.nmc-uk.org
- www.practicebasedlearning.org/home.htm
- www.learning-styles-online.com
- www.nmas.ac.uk/apply.html

Chapter 9

Reflection, Clinical Supervision and Portfolios

This chapter contains sections on reflection (the contents of which are probably not completely new to you), clinical supervision (as all registered nurses in the UK should be involved in this process), and portfolios and profiles. The last section is included as all registered nurses in the UK are required to create and maintain a portfolio and, within that, a profile outlining their career progression and identification of learning opportunities for the future.

Outcomes

On completion of this chapter you should be able to:

- describe the process of reflection, and exercise the skills required to carry this out;

- discuss the advantages of using reflection in practice;

- appreciate the concept and advantages of clinical supervision;

- have an understanding of the need to maintain a portfolio;

- appreciate the NMC's position on personal professional profiles;

- consider how you might structure your own portfolio.

REFLECTION

We're sure you have used the reflective process as a learning tool throughout your career, so this is just a reminder. Reflective practice is associated with learning from experience, and is viewed as an important strategy for health professionals who embrace life-long learning. There are many definitions in the literature of reflective practice and reflection. However, most agree that it is an active, conscious process where an experience is explored in order to gain new understandings and to learn something new. Reflection is often initiated when the individual practitioner encounters some problematic aspect of practice and attempts to make sense of it, and can be achieved either formally or informally. Peate (2006) believes the outcome may be the development of a deeper understanding of personal skills, enhanced self-awareness and individual learning needs. The NMC (2001) endorses reflection, stating that through reflection nurses can develop further and enhance their understanding of practice.

There are many different models for reflection, with no one being better than any other – which is used is a matter of personal choice, but the consensus from nursing literature is that reflection should be structured to enable learning to come as a result of it. Price (2002) suggests that reflection is more comfortable and effective if a step-by-step approach is used, and most of the reflective models acknowledge this with a broad outline of the stages being:

- thinking back over a situation;
- possibly discussing the incident with other people;
- re-evaluating the experience to seek possible new understandings;
- checking out new knowledge;
- developing an action plan for the future.

(Whitehead and Mason, 2003)

Good reflective practice underpins good professional practice in that reflection enables practitioners to review their progress and identify areas that have been successfully developed, and those that are in need of further development. It enhances a commitment to lifelong learning and continuous professional development (Somerset Academy, 2005).

MODELS OF REFLECTION

As mentioned above, there are many models of reflection to choose from. Outlined below are three of the most widely used models.

Gibbs' (1988) Reflective Cycle

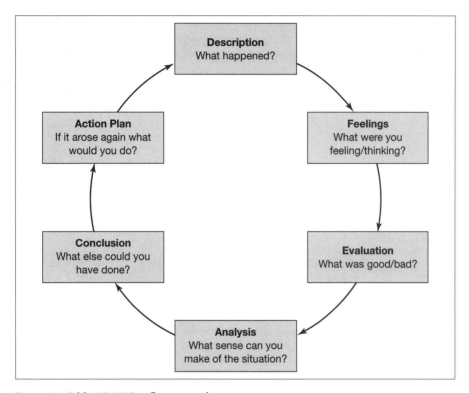

Figure 1 Gibbs' (1988) reflective cycle

Gibbs' (1988) reflective cycle (see Figure 1) is fairly straightforward and encourages a clear description of the situation, analysis of feelings, evaluation of the experience, analysis to make sense of the experience, a conclusion where other options are considered, and reflection upon the experience to examine what you would do if the situation arose again. This cycle can be used for reflective writing, as well as a basis for discussion. Jasper (2003) outlines the stages of Gibbs' cycle in greater detail and gives suggestions on how it should be used.

Stage 1: Description of the event

Describe in detail the event you are reflecting on. Include, for example: where were you; who else was there; why were you there; what were you doing; what were other people doing; what was the context of the event; what happened; what was your part in this; what parts did the other people play; what was the result?

Stage 2: Feelings

At this stage try to recall and explore the things that were going on inside your head – that is, why does this event stick in your mind? Include, for example: how were you feeling when the event started; what were you thinking about at the time; how did it make you feel; how did other people make you feel; how did you feel about the outcome of the event; what do you think about it now?

Stage 3: Evaluation

Try to evaluate or make a judgement about what happened. Consider what was good about the experience and what was bad about the experience, or what didn't go so well.

Stage 4: Analysis

Break the event down into its component parts so they can be explored separately. You may need to ask more detailed questions about the answers to the last stage. Include, for example: what went well; what did you do well; what did others do well; what went wrong or did not turn out how it should have done; in what way did you or others contribute to this?

Stage 5: Conclusion

This differs from the evaluation stage in that now you have explored the issue from different angles and have a lot of information on which to base your judgement. It is here that you are likely to develop insight into you own and other people's behaviour in terms of how it contributed to the outcome of the event. Remember the purpose of reflection is to learn from an experience. Without detailed analysis and the honest exploration that occurs during all the previous stages, it is unlikely that all aspects of the event will be taken into account and therefore valuable opportunities for learning can be missed. During this stage you should ask yourself what you could have done differently.

Stage 6: Action plan

During this stage you should think yourself forward into encountering the event again and to plan what you would do – would you act differently or would you be likely to do the same? Here the cycle is tentatively completed and suggests that, should the event occur again, it will be the focus of another reflective cycle.

Johns' (2002) Model for Structured Reflection: Version 13

Johns' (2002) model for structured reflection can be used as a guide for analysis of a critical incident or for general reflection on experience, and is useful for more complex analyses. Johns believes that the reflector should work with a supervisor, as he considers that through sharing reflections greater understanding of those experiences can be achieved, rather than the reflector undertaking a lone exercise. The stages of John's model of structured reflection are as follows.

- What issues seem significant to pay attention to?
- How was I feeling and what made me feel that way?
- What was I trying to achieve?
- Did I respond effectively and in tune with my values?
- What were the consequences of my action for the patient, others and myself?
- How were others feeling?
- What made them feel that way?
- What factors influenced the way I was feeling, thinking or responding?
- What knowledge did or might have informed me?
- To what extent did I act for the best?
- How does this situation connect with my previous experience?
- How might I respond more effectively given this situation again?
- What would be the consequences of alternative actions for the patient, others and myself?
- How do I now feel about this experience?
- Am I more able to support myself and others better as a consequence?
- Am I more available to work with patients, families and staff to help them meet their needs?

Stephenson's (1994) Reflective Model

Stephenson's reflective model is as follows.

- What was my role in this situation?
- Did I feel comfortable or uncomfortable? Why?
- What actions did I take?
- How did I and others act?
- Was it appropriate?
- How could I have improved the situation for myself, the patient, my mentor?
- What can I achieve in the future?
- Do I feel as if I have learnt anything new about myself?
- Did I expect anything different to happen? What and why?
- Has it changed my way of thinking in any way?

- What knowledge from theory and research can I apply to this situation?
- What broader issues, for example ethical, political or social, arise from this situation?
- What do I think about these broader issues?

(Stephenson, 1994, pp. 56–57)

Using reflective frameworks

As a summary to reflection, and regardless of which model for reflection is used, Price (2002) suggests that the challenge of using reflective frameworks is often in ensuring that you have considered the following.

- Did you consider your own prejudices?
- Did you avoid seeing only the familiar and/or one perspective?
- Did you consider what others might have intended to signal through their behaviour?
- Did you make use of and check out all the available information?
- Did you actually learn something new?
- Did you form an action plan for how to approach this differently in future?

Activity

Select a model of reflection and record a significant learning event from clinical practice. This could be included within your professional portfolio.

CLINICAL SUPERVISION

Clinical supervision is a term that has been used by registered nurses and other health care professionals to provide a purposeful, practice-focused relationship that enables the nurse to reflect on practice with the support of a skilled supervisor (Peate, 2006). It was introduced in the workplace for nurses during the 1990s, following the Department of Health's document *A Vision for the Future* (1993) as a way of using reflective practice and shared experiences as part of continuing professional development (CPD). The concept, however, has been long established in professions such as midwifery, social work, psychotherapy and counselling.

Clinical supervision has the support of the NMC, which states 'supervision aims to identify solutions to problems, improve practice and increase understanding of professional issues' (UKCC, 1996); and it fits well in the clinical governance framework by helping to ensure better and improving nursing practice (RCN, 2002). The Department of Health (Department of Health, 1993, p. 3) defines clinical supervision as:

A formal process of professional support and learning which enables individual practitioners to develop knowledge and competence, assume responsibility for their own practice and enhance consumer protection and safety in care in complex clinical situations.

The RCN (2002) and NMC (UKCC, 1996) believe that effective clinical supervision allows the practitioner to:

- reflect on nursing practice;
- identify room for improvement;
- develop expertise and promote standards of care;
- devise new ways of learning;
- gain professional support;
- develop a deeper understanding of professional issues;

Clinical supervision is different from any discussion you may have with your line manager in that it involves stepping back and reflecting on practice with a clinical supervisor who is external to your immediate workplace. It should not be confused with appraisal, development review or any other management activity. It is not a mandatory requirement from the NMC, and anything said in sessions should be confidential. Clinical supervision sessions must be carefully structured and managed with clearly defined aims and objectives. Ground rules and responsibilities should be clearly defined and there should be a contract of commitment from both supervisor and supervisees in order for it to be a meaningful exercise.

There are various models or approaches to clinical supervision: one-to-one supervision, group supervision, or peer group supervision. The choice of approach will depend upon a number of factors, including personal choice, access to supervision, length of experience, qualifications, availability of supervisory groups, etc. However, all partaking in clinical supervision will have a supervisor who is a skilled professional and assists other practitioners in the development of their skills, knowledge and professional values. Fitzgerald (2000, p. 155) believes that:

Within these types of supervisory relationships reflection plays an important role in the clinical supervision process. The use of a reflective framework facilitates a structured approach to the agenda of the supervisory meeting and helps maintain the focus on practice whilst enabling a questioning approach.

Driscoll (1994) agrees with this, but suggests that that not all reflective practice is clinical supervision, but potentially all good supervision is reflective practice. He also points out that clinical supervision is about reflecting not only on the big issues surrounding clinical practice but also on the seemingly insignificant and most ordinary of practice activities. Driscoll's (2000) model of clinical supervision is probably the most widely known and used. It is in the form of reflective practice, but the essential difference is that it involves another person(s) helping someone to reflect. It is cyclical in nature and is known as the WHAT? It contains three elements, these elements being used by a supervisee to prepare for clinical supervision:

- WHAT? – a description of the event;
- so WHAT? – an analysis of the event;
- now WHAT? – proposed actions following the event.

Driscoll (2000) also lists a number of trigger questions, which are not dissimilar to those posed by Johns (2002) and Stephenson (1994). In addition, he lists some skills and attributes required (of both supervisor and supervisee) for effective clinical supervision:

- a willingness to learn from what happens in practice;
- being open enough to share elements of practice with other people;
- being motivated enough to replay aspects of clinical practice;
- knowledge for clinical practice can emerge from within, as well as outside clinical practice;
- being aware of the conditions necessary for reflection to occur;
- a belief that it is possible to change as a practitioner;
- the ability to describe in detail before analysing practice problems;
- recognising the consequences of reflection;
- the ability to articulate what happens in practice;
- a belief that there is no end point about learning in practice;
- not being defensive about what other people notice about one's practice;
- being courageous enough to act on reflection;
- working out schemes to personally action what has been learned;
- being honest in describing clinical practice to others.

(Driscoll, 2000, p. 30)

Activity

Have you taken part in clinical supervision sessions? If so, reflect on how this process has helped your professional development.

PORTFOLIOS AND PROFILES

The NMC (2006a) states that all registered nurses in the UK are required to create and maintain a portfolio and, within that, a personal professional profile outlining their career progress and identifying learning opportunities for the future. You may be familiar with the concept of maintaining your own portfolio and, indeed, may have used your portfolio or profile when applying for a job. The following pages aim to outline the NMC's views on portfolio building, and the reasons why all registered nurses practising in the UK must undertake this activity. However, there is sometimes confusion as to what a profile is and what a portfolio is. Brown (1995) offers the following explanations.

- *A portfolio is* a personal, private collection of evidence which demonstrates the continuing acquisition of skills, knowledge, attitudes, understanding and achievements. It is both retrospective and prospective, as well as reflecting the current stage of development and activity of the individual.
- *A profile is* a collection of evidence which is selected from the personal portfolio for a particular purpose, and for the attention of a particular audience. Therefore an array of profiles can be developed to meet different needs, for example when applying for a job, for professional development review, etc.

Your profile

The NMC states on its website that a profile is:

> a record of career progress and professional development. It is not a CV, a daily diary of events or your whole life history! A profile is a flexible but comprehensive account of your professional development. However, it is more than a record of achievement. It is based on a regular process of reflection and recording what you learn from every day experiences, as well as planned learning activity. Your profile is your personal document. It does not belong to the NMC or your employer and its contents are private and confidential to you.
> **www.nmcuk.org/aArticle.aspx?ArticleID=330&Keyword=Personal%
> 20and%20professional%20and%20profile**

The profile has two key functions:

- contributing to your professional development by helping you to recognise and appreciate your abilities, achievements and experience;
- providing an information source on which you can draw in order to collect material about standards of education following registration.

Organising and documenting your information (NMC, 2006a)

There is no such thing as an official profile document and the NMC does not produce profile documents. Whatever format you choose – ring binder, box file, floppy disc or one of the profiles available commercially – the main factors should be flexibility, accessibility and confidentiality. You should be aware that your profile will contain personal information, so it should not be accessible to others without your permission. At the same time, you should not document any information which could identify patients, clients or carers as this could constitute a breach of confidentiality. For these reasons, you could consider dividing your profile into two sections – one containing confidential information and the other containing material that the NMC may require for audit purposes. As there is no definite format as to what should be included in a portfolio because it is personal to you, you might wish to consider the following as a guide:

- personal details – CV and employment record;
- educational and academic record;
- personal and professional development (past and present);
- professional work with key learning points;
- non-nursing experiences;
- future development.

Maintaining a profile will give you real benefits. It will:

- help you assess your current standards of practice;
- develop your analytical skills through reflection on what you do;
- enable you to review and evaluate past experience and learning to help you plan for the future;
- provide effective and current information if you apply for a job or a course;
- demonstrate experiential learning which may allow you to obtain credit towards further qualifications.

Boud *et al* (1985) give guidelines or tips on how to develop and maintain a portfolio which may be of help:

- seek out a method which suits you – it is important to keep your portfolio personal – write about what is important for you, not what others say you should;
- be frank, honest and spontaneous in your entries – use your own words, say what you feel;
- have a positive approach when writing – write regularly and stick at it;
- feel free to express yourself in diagrams, pictures or other types of material;

- a portfolio is meant to be a workbook – work through entries a number of times, go back to early entries and further reflect on them;
- focus on things that are important – do not waste time on trivialities;
- do not be rigid in the way you keep your portfolio – be prepared to change your methods;
- record experiences as soon as possible after they happen, and in as much detail as possible;
- important issues may need to be shared with others and feedback recorded – this will deepen your understanding of situations.

(Adapted from Boud *et al*, 1985)

As previously mentioned, *The PREP Handbook* (NMC, 2006a) outlines the standards which nurses must achieve in order to re-register every three years. One of the requirements is that nurses must have undertaken and recorded their continuing professional development (CPD) and must reflect on how it has influenced their practice. Although the NMC states that that it is entirely up to individual nurses how they achieve the standard, the expectation is that this is recorded in a personal professional profile (PPP).

Activity

Referring to *The PREP Handbook* (NMC 2006a, pp. 10–11), reflect on a learning activity you have undertaken recently and complete the following activity. You may like to use the headings the NMC set out.

- *The nature of the learning activity* – Briefly describe the learning activity, for example, reading a relevant clinical article, attending a course, observing practice. State how many hours this took.
- *Description of learning activity* – Describe what the learning activity actually consisted of – include, for example, why you decided to do the learning activity or how the opportunity came about; where, when and how you did the learning activity; the type of learning activity, and what you expected to gain from it.
- *Outcome of the learning activity* – Give a personal view of how the learning informed and influenced your work – what effect has this learning had on the way in which you work, or intend to work in the future? Do you have any ideas or plans for follow-up learning? The way in which this learning has influenced my work is …

Chapter 10

Medicine, IV Fluid and Blood Administration

The aim of this chapter is to outline the considerations you need to make when administering oral medications, giving intravenous (IV) fluids or transfusing blood to patients in the UK. Employers will outline policies about medicine administration (drug rounds) and intravenous medications, and nurses are expected to undertake an assessment of competence (set by the employer) prior to administering any medicines in clinical practice. In some instances this will include administration of intravenous fluids and blood transfusions. The following pages should act as a reminder and help you study for these assessments.

Outcomes

On completion of this chapter you should be able to:

- discuss the legal and professional responsibilities of the registered nurse when administering medications, intravenous therapy and blood transfusions;

- describe the actions necessary when administering medicines, intravenous fluids and blood;

- discuss potential complications, and subsequent actions taken, in administering medicines and blood transfusions;

- display numeracy skills by accurately calculating medicine dosages and intravenous rates.

INTRODUCTION

A prescribed medicine is the most common treatment provided for patients in the NHS (Peate, 2006). If anything goes wrong with the administration of that medicine the nurse is accountable in the criminal courts, the civil courts, before their employer and before the NMC (Dimond, 2005).

As previously identified, the NMC issues the *Code of Professional Conduct* (NMC, 2004a) to all practitioners. In addition, it issues *Guidelines for the Administration of Medicines* (2004b) and, while this guidance has no legal force in itself, it establishes principles for safe practice in the management and administration of medicines by registered nurses in the UK (Dimond, 2005). The *Guidelines for the Administration of Medicines* (NMC, 2004b, p. 3) state:

> The administration of medicines is an important aspect of the professional practice of persons whose names are on the Council's register. It is not solely a mechanistic task to be performed in strict compliance with the written prescription of a medical practitioner. It requires thought and the exercise of professional judgement ... .

Activity

Referring to Chapter 2: Legal, Professional and Ethical Issues, describe three circumstances where you, as a registered nurse, could be judged negligent in respect of administering medicines.

LEGISLATION CONCERNING MEDICINES

The *London Pharmacopoeia* listing approved drugs was first published in 1618, but the control of medicines in Britain can be traced back to the fifteenth century. In the nineteenth century the Pharmaceutical Society of Great Britain was formed and legislation introduced to regulate the sale of poisons. The creation of the NHS in 1948 led to the setting up of a government committee to consider the value of medicines, but it was not until the 1960s that a government White Paper on the safety and quality of medications led to the introduction of legislation to cover all aspects of medication management. The need for this legislation was compounded by the Thalidomide tragedy, when a medication prescribed for morning sickness, caused congenital malformations when given in the first trimester of pregnancy. Today, the legislation in the UK controlling manufacture, supply, storage and administration of medicines consists of the Medicines Act 1968, the Misuse of Drugs Act 1971, Misuse of Drugs Regulations 2001 and various statutory instruments. Other legislation you need to consider when practising in the UK includes:

- the Misuse of Drugs Act (Safe Custody) Regulations 1973 SI 1973 as amended by Misuse of Drugs Regulations 2001;
- NMC's *Guidelines for the Administration of Medicines* (2004b);
- NMC's *Code of Professional Conduct* (2004a);
- the Care Standards Act 2000. The Care Standards Act came into force in 2002. Its intention was to regulate the private care industry to meet the same standards nationally. The National Minimum Standards provide direction in meeting these standards and are also used to benchmark performance within the inspection process by the Commission for Social Care Inspection.

Medicines Act 1968 (from Dimond, 2005)

This Act set up a comprehensive system of medicine controls covering:

- administrative system;
- licensing system;
- retail pharmacies;
- packing and labelling of medicinal products;
- British pharmacopoeia;
- the sale and supply of medicines to the public:
  - prescription-only medicines (POMs) – these are medicines that may be supplied or administered to a patient only on the instruction of an appropriate practitioner (a doctor, dentist or nurse prescriber);
  - pharmacy-only medicines – these can be purchased from a registered primary care pharmacy, provided that the sale is supervised by the pharmacist;
  - general sale list medicines (GSLs) – these do not need either a prescription or the supervision of a pharmacist and can be obtained from retail outlets (for example supermarkets).

Misuse of Drugs Act 1971

Controlled drugs are defined in the Misuse of Drugs Act 1971. They include those drugs which are habit-forming and certain other narcotics that have a profound effect on the central nervous system. The Act:

- lists and classifies controlled drugs;
- creates criminal offences in relation to the manufacture, supply and possession of controlled drugs;
- gives the Secretary of State power to make regulations and directions to prevent misuse of controlled drugs;
- creates an advisory council on misuse of drugs;
- gives powers of search, arrest and forfeiture.

Further information can be obtained from the Medicines and Healthcare Products Regulatory Agency (MHRA) at **www.mhra.gov.uk**

ADMINISTRATION OF MEDICINES

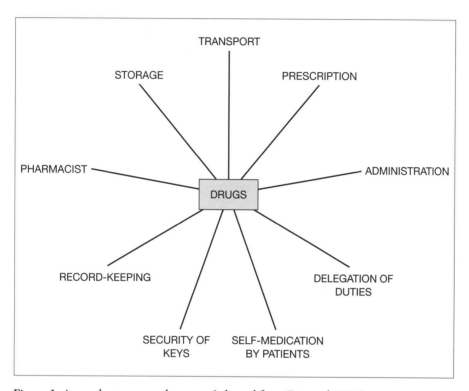

Figure 1 Areas that concern the nurse (adapted from Dimond, 2005)

While you are practising in the UK there are many aspects of medicine administration that you, as a registered nurse, need to be aware of. Dimond (2005) suggests the main areas of concern are those shown in Figure 1. Some of these headings are explored more fully in the next few pages, whereas others may be found in *Guidelines for the Administration of Medicines* (NMC, 2004b).

Prescription

There are several ways that medicines are prescribed in the UK. Generally a doctor or qualified nurse prescriber is responsible for patient diagnosis and initiation of medicine treatment, and can order medicines and controlled drugs (depending on local policy for nurse prescribers). The prescriptions they write must include:

- the patient's full name, date of birth, weight and allergies;
- the generic (proper) name of the medicine (not the trade name), strength, dose, form (elixir, tabs, etc.), route of administration and frequency to be taken;
- a signature and date by the doctor/nurse prescriber.

The prescription must be indelible and legible. It should also state the duration of the course of medication before a patient review should take place.

Telephone (verbal) orders for a prescription (NMC, 2007)

An instruction by telephone to administer a previously unprescribed medicine is not acceptable. In exceptional circumstances, where a medication has been previously prescribed and the prescriber is unable to issue a new prescription, but where changes in the dose are considered necessary, the use of IT (e.mail or fax) is the preferred method. This must be followed up by a new prescription confirming the changes within a given time period (usually 24 hours). Each hospital or care home will have a policy about taking telephone orders, and it is your responsibility as a registered nurse to become conversant with them in your clinical area.

Nurse prescribing

Primary legislation permitting nurse prescribing is set out in the Medicinal Products: Prescription by Nurses, Midwives and Health Visitors Act 1992, which was implemented in 1994. This enabled district nurses and health visitors who had undertaken an accredited Extended Nurse Prescribing Programme to prescribe medications from the Nurse Prescribers' Formulary. Since then, additional legislation and amendments have widened the numbers and categories of nurses who can prescribe.

> If you wish to know more about nurse prescribing access the NMC Website at **www.nmc-uk.org** and read the position statement.

Patient Group Directions (PGDs)

Patient Group Directions (PGDs) have been in existence since August 2000. A PGD is a written instruction for the supply and/or administration of medicines to certain groups of patients that fit certain criteria within the directions; without the need for a prescription or an instruction from a pre-scriber. PDGs are drawn up locally by doctors (or dentists, pharmacists or other health care professionals), and *must* be signed by either a doctor or dentist *and* a pharmacist. A PGD is not a form of prescribing and, unlike prescribing, health care professionals entitled to work with a PGD do not require any additional formal qualification. However, employers have a responsibility to ensure that only fully competent, trained health care pro-fessionals use PGDs, and may specify local training and assessment of competence. PGDs cannot be delegated and the same nurse or health care practitioner must both supply and administer the medicine. PDGs are not appropriate where a range of different medicines need to be administered at the same time. Prior to April 2003, only NHS organisations could use PGDs, but legislation now allows a range of non-NHS organisations to use them.

The pharmacist

In the UK the pharmacist is legally responsible for the supply and distribu-tion of drugs in accordance with the law. However, in some cases, nurses who have had additional training, and in line with the hospital policy where they work *and* with the written instructions of a medical practi-tioner, may dispense medicines. The role of a pharmacist also includes that of a resource person for medicine information, and they are responsible for checking that any newly prescribed medicine will not interact dangerously with, or nullify any existing medication. All medicines must be clearly and concisely labelled and should describe the contents including:

- the patient's name;
- the name of the drug;
- the strength;
- the dose;
- the frequency;
- any special instructions (such as storage, precautions, etc.);
- the dispensing date (expiry date if appropriate).

If the label appears to have been tampered with or altered in any way it must be reported and returned to the pharmacy immediately.

The responsibility for storing medications also lies with the pharmacist, in conjunction with the senior nurse (ward manager) in a hospital setting, or with the manager and senior nurse in a private institution. The responsibility for administration of medicines lies with individual registered nurses. All medicines must be kept in locked cupboards. Individual medicines and some stock items can be held in a mobile medicine trolley and, when this trolley is not in use, it must be secured to a wall by a locking device, or kept within a locked cupboard.

Activity

Look up three drugs you have administered in the past. What are the potential side effects/contra-indications for these medications? Are there any drugs they are incompatible with? Make a few notes. You might like to register at the website of eBNF at **www.bnf.org** (it's free!) or use **http://emc.medicines.org.uk**

The nurse's role in the administration of medicines

Medicines must be administered according to the patient's individual needs and in accordance with national, professional and local policies. When administrating any medicine a registered nurse must (NMC, 2004b):

- know the therapeutic uses of the medicine to be administered, its normal dosage, side effects, precautions and contra-indications;
- be certain of the identity of the patient to whom the medicine is to be administered;
- check that the prescription, or the label on the medicine dispensed by a pharmacist, is clearly written and unambiguous;
- have considered the dosage, method of administration, route and timing of the administration in the context of the condition of the patient and co-existing therapies – this is often abbreviated into the five Rs:
  - right drug;
  - right dose;
  - right route;
  - right time;
  - right patient;
- check the expiry date of the medication to be administered;
- check that the patient is not allergic to the medication before administering it;
- contact the prescriber or another authorised prescriber without delay where contra-indications to the prescribed medication are discovered, where the patient develops a reaction to the medication, or where assessment of the patient indicates that the medication is no longer suitable;
- make a clear, accurate and immediate record of all medication administered, intentionally withheld or refused by the patient, ensuring

that any written entries and the signature are clear and legible – it is also your responsibility to ensure that a record is made when delegating the task of administering medication;

- where supervising a student nurse in the administration of medicines, clearly countersign the signature of the student.

Prior to any medicine being administered in a health care setting in the UK, the following must be on the prescription chart, which must be clearly and indelibly written, typed or computer generated:

- patient's name;
- weight if dosage of medication is related to patient's weight;
- medication prescribed by the proper (not generic) name;
- strength of drug;
- dose of medication;
- frequency of administration;
- route of administration;
- start and finish dates;
- signature and date by the authorised prescriber.

Covert administration of medicines

Disguising medication in the absence of informed consent of the patient may be regarded as deception and, if you undertake this practice, you must be convinced that you are doing this in the patient's best interests and be aware you are accountable for this action. The NMC (2007) states that covert medicine administration should be performed only in life-saving circumstances or to prevent the deterioration of a patient's condition, or to ensure improvement in a patient's physical or mental health. As a registered nurse you must be assured that you have the support (or otherwise) of the rest of the multiprofessional team for covertly administering medicines, and this should be recorded. Each organisation involved in health care should have a policy or protocol on covert administration of medicines and you should be familiar with the one in your clinical area.

Crushing medication

Many patients are unable to swallow tablets or capsules whole, and the crushing or opening of capsules is often a method used to administer medication to such patients. However, in doing this you may alter the chemical properties of the medication. There are also legal issues surrounding the crushing of tablets (NMC, 2007):

- the crushing of a tablet, in most cases, renders its use 'unlicensed' – consequently the manufacturer may assume no liability for any ensuing harm that may come to the patient or the person administering it;
- under the Medicines Act 1968, only medical and dental practitioners can authorise the administration of 'unlicensed' medicines, therefore it is illegal to crush a tablet before administration without the authorisation of the prescriber;
- when an 'unlicensed' medicine is authorised to be administered a percentage of the liability for any harm that might ensue will lie with the administering nurse.

Therefore, if your patient is unable to swallow tablets, an alternative such as a liquid should be prescribed instead. If there is no alternative preparation of the medication, then crushing should take place only following consultation with the prescriber and pharmacist, and this must be recorded.

Self-administration

Some clinical areas have adopted a policy for self-administration of medicines and, if this is the case, an internal policy will exist concerning this. As with all policies, you need to become familiar with its content before taking part in this procedure. The NMC (2004b, p. 4) reminds nurses that overseeing self-administration of medicines by patients is just as important a procedure as administering them yourself:

> In administering any medication, or assisting or overseeing self-administration of medication, you must exercise your personal judgement and apply your knowledge and skill in the given situation.

The registered nurse has a responsibility to the patient who is self-administering to ensure that they are aware of the medicines they are taking, the correct dosages and possible side effects to look for.

Controlled drugs

Controlled drugs are defined in the Misuse of Drugs Act 1971. They include those drugs which are habit-forming and certain other narcotics which have a profound effect on the central nervous system.

Custody of controlled drugs

Controlled drugs must be kept in a locked safe or receptacle within a locked cupboard with a warning light to show when the cupboard is open. The policy for safe custody and administration of controlled drugs is clearly laid down in policies that all nurses are responsible for reading and understanding.

Disposal of medicines

In NHS establishments all medicines no longer required or that are out of date must be returned to the pharmacy. In care homes disposal of unwanted medication is via a clinical waste company. In any establishment only single doses of medicines that are not administered for any reason may be disposed of down a sluice or toilet system. A single dose of a controlled drug which requires destruction may be disposed of in a sluice or toilet system, but two people, one of whom must be a registered nurse, must witness the disposal and enter the fact in the Controlled Drug Register.

Further reading

Further information about medicine administration can be found on the NMC website (**www.nmc-uk.org**) – type 'medicines management' into the A–Z of advice.

PRINCIPLES OF PRACTICE

While no one likes to make a mistake when administering medicines, unfortunately mistakes do happen. However, by following correct procedures, the opportunity for mistakes can lessen, and the following pages explore what an error is, and how 'best practice' can be promoted. A medication error can be defined as a preventable prescribing, dispensing or administration error (Cooper, 1995). Errors may be made by:

- doctors;
- pharmacists;
- nurses;
- health care assistants;
- any other health care professional involved with medication.

A medication error occurs when:

- the wrong medication is administered;
- the wrong patient is administered the medication;
- the patient receives an over- or under-dose;
- a dose is missed or late;
- the medication chart is not signed;
- the medication is changed from its licensed formulation (for example, it has been dissolved in tea).

It has been stated that over 90 per cent of errors may not be reported (the *Society Guardian*, 2000). There are many reasons for this but perhaps the key two are not realising an error has been made, or fear of the outcome if an error is declared. A 'no-blame' culture is currently advocated as the best approach when managing any error in the workplace (NMC, 2004b). This is encouraged to ensure prompt reporting for the well being of both patient and staff, and ensuring that learning takes place from the error made so that it does not happen again. Therefore, all errors and incidents must be investigated taking full account of the context and circumstances.

Preventing errors

In some instances there may be an argument that it is not the individual nurse responsible for administering medicines, but the working environment, that causes the incidence of error to increase. A common example of this is being interrupted during the medicine round. By using the approach that it is a 'team concern' it may be easier to explore how errors can be prevented. In this way the culture of the workplace can move from one that manages mistakes to one that proactively works to eliminate or to minimise the risk of error.

Principles of best practice can be identified as points of safety. That is, if all possibilities are considered, the risk can be significantly reduced or eliminated. These can be listed under three headings:

1 *Knowledge:*

- be aware of correct storage, expiration dates, labelling, etc.;
- know therapeutic dosages, side effects, contra-indications, precautions;
- be aware of where to obtain information;
- consider dosage, timing and route in context with patient history.

2 *Communication:*

- ensure clear record-keeping;
- ensure appropriate and clearly written prescriptions;
- ensure allergies are clearly written and appropriate persons are informed;
- ensure patient consent and understanding, whenever possible;
- be aware of the patient's care plan.

3 *Procedure:*

- ensure clear procedure that is understood by all staff;
- ensure patient identity;
- ensure that policies for complete medication management are known to all and regularly reviewed;
- ensure that patients are regularly reviewed and relevant persons notified when a reaction is noted or treatment no longer appears effective.

HYPERSENSITIVITY TO MEDICINES

As a registered nurse you will already be aware of the adverse reactions to medicines that patients may experience. These include the side effects of the medicine, intolerance or excess effects of a normal dose of the medicine, and hypersensitivity to the medicine. As a way of a reminder the following pages outline the features of an anaphylactic reaction and the European Resuscitation Council's guidelines (which are used throughout the UK) for treatment of anaphylaxis (see Figure 2).

Anaphylactic reactions vary in severity and progress may be rapid or slow and, rarely, manifestations may be delayed by a few hours or persist for more than 24 hours. Clinical features include:

- angio-oedema;
- urticaria;
- dyspnoea;
- hypotension;
- acute irreversible asthma or laryngeal oedema;
- rhinitis;
- conjunctivitis;
- abdominal pain;
- vomiting;
- diarrhoea;
- sense of impending doom;
- skin colour – either flushed or pale;
- cardiovascular collapse.

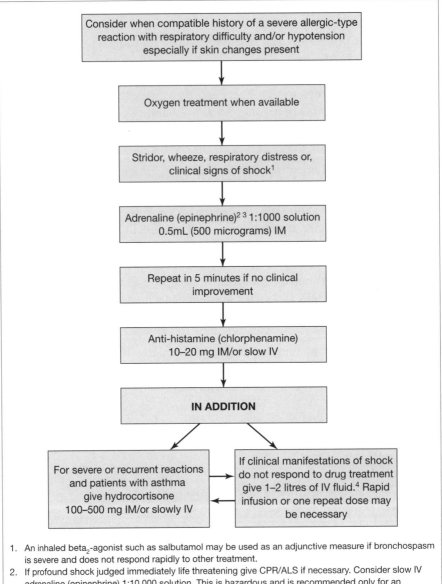

Consider when compatible history of a severe allergic-type reaction with respiratory difficulty and/or hypotension especially if skin changes present

Oxygen treatment when available

Stridor, wheeze, respiratory distress or, clinical signs of shock[1]

Adrenaline (epinephrine)[2 3] 1:1000 solution 0.5mL (500 micrograms) IM

Repeat in 5 minutes if no clinical improvement

Anti-histamine (chlorphenamine) 10–20 mg IM/or slow IV

IN ADDITION

For severe or recurrent reactions and patients with asthma give hydrocortisone 100–500 mg IM/or slowly IV

If clinical manifestations of shock do not respond to drug treatment give 1–2 litres of IV fluid.[4] Rapid infusion or one repeat dose may be necessary

1. An inhaled beta$_2$-agonist such as salbutamol may be used as an adjunctive measure if bronchospasm is severe and does not respond rapidly to other treatment.
2. If profound shock judged immediately life threatening give CPR/ALS if necessary. Consider slow IV adrenaline (epinephrine) 1:10,000 solution. This is hazardous and is recommended only for an experienced practitioner who can also obtain IV access without delay. Note the different strength of adrenaline (epinephrine) that may be required for IV use.
3. If adults are treated with an adrenaline auto-injection the 300 micrograms will usually be sufficient. A second dose may be required. Half doses of adrenaline (epinephrine) may be safer for patients on amitriptyline, micramine, or beta blocker.
4. A crystalicid may be safer than a colloid.

Figure 2 Anaphylactic reactions: treatment algorithm for adults by first medical responders (European Resuscitation Council, 2005)

Case study

Read the following article and then identify and comment on the clauses of the *Code of Professional Conduct* (NMC, 2004a) and the *Guidelines for the Administration of Medicines* (NMC, 2004a) that David breached. (This article is reproduced with permission from *The British Journal of Nursing*.)

STAFF NURSE REMOVED FROM NURSING REGISTER FOR MIS-MANAGEMENT OF DRUG ROUNDS

British Journal of Nursing, 2005, 14: 953: Professional Misconduct Series

David was a staff nurse employed by a large hospital trust in the north of England. He usually worked night duty and was known for his efficiency in completing nursing tasks.

The ward David worked on contained many older patients, who were recovering from various medical interventions. Debra, who was a new staff nurse came to work opposite shifts with David and could not believe how quickly he completed his drug rounds. One day she thought she discovered the reason why this was so: she found out that one of David's patients had been signed off as receiving his drugs when in fact he had not received them.

This came to light over a weekend when it was difficult to obtain certain drugs as the pharmacy was closed. Debra remembered giving the last dose of a drug to a patient and then putting the empty container on the pharmacy trolley. When she followed on from David again she was surprised to note that David had signed off as having given the drug which she had previously sent back empty to the pharmacy. At first Debra thought David may have found another stock of the drug, but when she checked again this appeared to be untrue.

When she challenged David about the incident he shrugged it off by saying that he had signed the prescription chart before he had checked the stock. He apologised for the oversight and gave an assurance that there would be no further errors on his part.

Debra accepted David's explanation and decided not to take any further action. Unfortunately when Debra carried a drug round a few days later she found two pots in the medicine trolley, both of which contained supposedly dispensed medication. One pot contained dispensed temazepam syrup, which she identified because of the distinctive smell, and the other pot contained two tablets of MST 10mg, which she recognised from the size and colour.

When asked why he had not administered the MST, David replied that he had no idea, adding that he might have been called away and had then forgotten. David also said that he left the temazepam in the trolley to remind him that he had not administered it. Debra mentioned this to the senior nurse, who arranged for David to undertake a training session regarding the procedures for the administration of medicines.

When Debra came to undertake a monthly drug count and audit of medicines she found that there were unexplained surpluses of medication, particularly for the patients who were more confused. Debra wrote in her statement that she had returned the surplus stock to the pharmacy during the previous month and was surprised therefore, that the discrepancies were so large.

Shortly after this incident when David was on duty another discrepancy occurred. This involved large quantities of medication being checked and found exactly as they were the previous evening. A seal on a new bottle of Alupent was intact despite it being prescribed for a patient. David claimed that the reason for the same levels was that he borrowed medication for other patients. Unfortunately he was unable to identify whose medication he had borrowed and could not remember why it had been necessary for him to borrow another patient's medication when that patient's medication was also in the drug trolley.

When asked about the other patients who had been signed off as receiving their medications yet the stock levels were the same, he replied that he did not know why he had not administered the medication.

David's case was referred to the NMC, where he reiterated that he could not explain why he did not give the patients their medications. One possible excuse was that he had been suffering from stress since his divorce. David was not referred to the health committee but admitted that he could not give a reasonable explanation for his actions. He was charged on 10 counts of making errors in the administration of drugs and his name was removed from the register for a minimum of five years.

Note: this case is in a series based on actual cases that were reported to the NMC. They were complied by George Castledine, Professor and Consultant of General Nursing, University of Central England, Birmingham, and Dudley Group of Hospitals NHS Trust.

INTRAVENOUS THERAPY

Most UK employers assess nurses prior to letting them administer intravenous fluids so, again, this section is a reminder of those things you need to consider when undertaking this procedure, and to help you with any assessment you may have to take. Nurses play a crucial role in the management of IV therapy and the prevention or early detection of complications (Dougherty and Lamb, 1999). Depending on the solutions used, and the condition of the patient, IV therapy may be continuous, intermittent or as a single dose injection. It can be administered via either a peripheral cannula or central catheter, however peripheral venous cannulation is the commonest method used for intravenous therapy (Waitt *et al*, 2004).

Indications for peripheral venous cannulation

These are:

- intravenous fluids;
- limited parenteral nutrition;
- blood and blood products;
- drug administration (continuous or intermittent);
- prophylactic use before procedures;
- prophylactic use in unstable patients.

Contra-indications and cautions for peripheral venous cannulation

These are:

- inflammation or infection of the insertion site;
- forearm veins in patients with renal failure (may be needed for arteriovenous fistulae);
- irritant drugs into small veins with low flow rates (that is, leg and foot veins).

Crystalloids and colloids

There are two types of fluids that are used for intravenous infusions: crystalloids and colloids. Crystalloids are aqueous solutions of mineral salts or other water-soluble molecules, whereas colloids contain larger, insoluble molecules, such as gelatin. Blood itself is a colloid. The most commonly used crystalloid fluid is normal saline, a solution of sodium chloride at 0.9 per cent concentration, which is close to the concentration in the blood. Ringer's lactate is another isotonic solution often used for large-volume fluid replacement. A solution of 5 per cent dextrose in water is often used if the patient is at risk for having low blood sugar or high sodium. The choice of fluids may also depend on the chemical properties of any medications being given.

Choice of administration (giving) set

- Blood set – for blood and blood products with integral filter.
- Solution set – standard administration set for most fluids.
- Burette set – for more accurate fluid delivery and in children.

Peripheral cannulae should be changed routinely after 48–72 hours (Waitt *et al*, 2004) as the rate of phlebitis increases with time.

Managing the infusion site (Dougherty and Lamb, 1999)

Observation of the site

The cannula site should be inspected at least once a day and every time IV drugs are administered. Observe for redness (phlebitis, thrombophlebitis), heat (infection) and swelling (extravasation or infiltration). The insertion site should not be painful.

Types of dressing

The peripheral IV site should be covered with a dressing that is sterile, easy to apply and remove. This keeps the site free from exogenous infection, secures the cannula in place and allows easy visual inspection of the site. It should be changed only if the dressing becomes wet or bloodstained or haemoserous fluid collects around the site.

Prevention of contamination

Asepsis is the key preventative measure in reducing the likelihood of infection, and hand washing is the most important aspect of this. Prior to any manipulation of the cannula, IV fluid, administration set, IV site or change of dressing, thorough hand washing must take place and, in most instances, sterile gloves be worn (check your employer's policy). Minimal handling of the administration system will also help prevent infection.

Methicillin-resistant Staphylococcus Aureus (MRSA)

Methicillin-resistant Staphylococcus aureus (MRSA) is a strain of Staphylococcus aureus which is resistant to methicillin and other antibiotics, and this resistance has been evident for the last 40 years (RCN,

2005). It colonises the skin, particularly the nose, skin folds, hairline, perineum and navel and commonly survives in these areas without causing infection. The patient becomes clinically infected only if the organism invades the skin or deeper tissues and multiplies. Transmission is by person-to-person contact or via equipment, and a working party in 1998 found that MRSA was prevalent in patients with intravenous devices. The symptoms are the same as for any infection and include redness, swelling and tenderness at the site of infection. In order to reduce the spread of MRSA nurses should ensure (RCN, 2005):

- hand washing before and after contact with every patient or potentially contaminated equipment;
- hand washing after removal of gloves;
- keeping the environment as clean and dry as possible;
- thorough cleaning and drying of all equipment after use.

Further reading

Further information about infection control in general can be found on the NMC A–Z of advice website (**www.nmc-uk.org**). The links at the end of the infection control section are very helpful.

Intravenous fluids

All fluid to be infused should be checked and inspected prior to use as an aid to prevent contamination/infection and, if there is any doubt, the fluid should be returned to the pharmacy. Also:

- check the packaging is intact;
- inspect the container for punctures, air bubbles, discolouration, haziness and particles;
- check the expiry date of the fluid;
- record the batch number.

Infusion devices / pumps

An infusion device is designed to deliver measured amounts of drug or fluid (either intravenously or subcutaneously) over a period of time. It is set at an appropriate rate to achieve a desired therapeutic response (Richards and Edwards, 2003).

Gravity controllers

A gravity controller is a mechanical device that operates by gravity without pumping action. A detector is placed on the drip chamber to count the drops, with an automatic clamping mechanism to control the flow. The desired flow is set in drops per minute. Gravity controllers are used where volumetric accuracy is less important (Auty, 1995).

Volumetric pumps

Volumetric pumps are used when a large volume of fluid needs to be administered (for example, for parenteral nutrition). They work by calculating the volume delivered with the rate selected in millilitres per hour (Auty, 1995), and are capable of accurate delivery over a wide range of flow rates.

Syringe pumps

These are low-volume, high-accuracy devices designed to infuse at low flow rates where the rate is controlled by the drive speed of the piston attached to the syringe plunger (Auty, 1995). They are useful where small volumes of concentrated drugs need to be infused.

Patient Controlled Analgesia (PCA) pumps

These are also syringe pumps but their distinguishing feature is that they can deliver doses on demand, when the patient pushes a button. Doses can be limited to a designated maximum amount. This method of delivering analgesia increases patient satisfaction as less sedation is required.

Complications of intravenous therapy

Complications of intravenous therapy include:

- infection;
- extravasation;
- phlebitis;
- thrombophlebitis;
- precipitation;
- air embolus;
- circulation overload;
- speed shock.

Activity

Listed above are some complications of intravenous therapy. List and make notes about the recognition and management of these complications.

BLOOD TRANSFUSION

Along with assessing nurses on the administration of medicines and intravenous fluids, some UK employers also ask nurses to undertake assessment in the management of blood transfusions. A reminder of some of the information you may be assessed on is given in the following few pages.

A blood transfusion is defined as the administration of whole blood or any of its components to correct or treat a clinical abnormality (Mallett and Doherty, 2000). The first blood transfusion is reported to have been in 1492 when Pope Innocent was given the blood of three Roman citizens – unfortunately all of them died. In the centuries that followed the technique developed, the key milestone being in 1901 when Karl Landsteiner discovered that not all blood was the same and developed the ABO blood grouping that is used universally today. The Rhesus system was discovered in 1940.

Managing the transfusion

Filters

Blood must be administered through a blood administration set as it has an integral filter to remove red-cell debris, leucocytes, platelets and fibrin strands that clump together. There should be no need to use additional filters unless the patient is receiving multiple units or cardiac bypass surgery.

Checking procedures

Minimum checks must include:

- patient identification – name, date of birth, hospital number;
- blood identification – correct blood product, blood unit number against transfusion request form, expiry date, patient and donor blood group and Rhesus status;
- prior to transfusion check baseline observations of temperature, pulse, respiration and blood pressure;
- repeat observations at 30 minute intervals;
- change infusion set after two units of blood;
- each unit of blood should be transfused within five hours.

Transfusion reactions

The transfusion of any blood product carries with it the potential of a transfusion reaction which could be immediate or delayed.

Acute haemolytic reaction

Acute haemolytic reaction is directly related to incompatibilities in the ABO blood group system. For example, when blood containing anti-A antibodies (group B) mixes with blood containing A antigens (group A) the donor antibodies attach to the surface of the recipient's red blood cells, causing cells to clump together. Eventually these clumped cells can plug small blood vessels leading to disseminated intravascular coagulation. This antibody/antigen reaction activates a process that promotes and accelerates red-blood-cell destruction, which in turn causes free haemoglobin to be released into the blood stream. This damages the kidney tubules and can lead to renal failure and death. Reactions can occur after as little as 5ml of blood being transfused, and are almost wholly preventable as reactions result from incorrect blood cross-matching, clerical error or checking errors at the bedside (Mallet and Doherty, 2000).

- *Features* of an acute haemolytic reaction include: hypotension, pyrexia, chills, agitation, pain at the cannula site, lumbar pain, facial flushing, bleeding from wound sites and chest pain.
- *Action:* stop the infusion immediately. Treat hypotension and give appropriate therapy for disseminated intravascular coagulation.

Anaphylactic reactions

Anaphylactic reactions are rare and are usually due to the production of antibodies by patients who have had a previous blood transfusion. The antibodies in plasma combine with antigens in donated red blood cells, causing histamine to be released, which in turn causes an acute anaphylactic reaction. The risk of this can be lessened by transfusing packed cells where 80 per cent of the plasma (where the antibodies circulate) has been removed.

- *Features* of anaphylaxis include: angio-oedema, urticaria, dyspnoea, hypotension, acute irreversible asthma or laryngeal oedema, rhinitis, conjunctivitis, abdominal pain, vomiting, diarrhoea, sense of impending doom, skin colour – either flushed or pale, cardiovascular collapse.
- *Action:* stop the infusion and resuscitate patient.

Pyogenic reaction

Pyogenic reaction is probably the most common cause of fever and is not considered serious. Pyogens are the breakdown material from bacteria in blood before sterilisation.

- *Features* include pyrexia, but without signs of shock, followed by the pyrexia subsiding if the transfusion is slowed.

MEDICINE CALCULATION

'Mathematical accuracy is a matter of life and death in clinical nursing' (Keighley, 1984, cited in Cheung, 1986) – an old reference, but certainly one that is still relevant. Drug errors account for 25 per cent of all litigation claims against the NHS (Wright, 2005) and improving the drug calculation skills of nurses is one strategy identified by the Department of Health (2004b) to try to reduce this number by 40 per cent. The Department of Health (2004b) also states that medication errors are costing the NHS between £200 and £400 million per year. *Guidelines for Administration of Medicines* (NMC, 2004b, p. 7) states:

> Some drug administrations can require complex calculations to ensure that the correct volume or quantity of medication is administered. In these situations, it may be necessary for a second practitioner to check the calculation in order to minimise the risk of error. The use of calculators to determine volume or quantity of medication should not act as a substitute for arithmetical knowledge and skill.

Drug dosages

To calculate drug dosages and intravenous infusion rates requires competence in the use of both fractions and decimals. The formulae suggested are calculated in fractions, while the end result must be in decimals for administration. However, with calculating drugs dosages a certain amount of logic is also required – nurses should be encouraged to predict mentally what the answer might be. For example, the dose ordered is Chlorphenamine 3 mg. The stock dose is 2 mg in 5 ml. Is the answer going to be greater or less than 5 ml?

Fractions

Simplifying or cancelling down fractions:

To simplify a fraction, divide the top and bottom figures by a common factor (a number that will go into both). For example:

$$\frac{25}{75} = \frac{1}{3} \qquad \text{Both figures have been divided by 25.}$$

This calculation may be done in more than one step:

$$\frac{25}{75} \text{ (both divided by 5)} = \frac{5}{15} \text{ (both divided by 5)} = \frac{1}{3}$$

Activity

Simplify the following fractions:

1a $\dfrac{12}{28}$ 1b $\dfrac{8}{12}$ 1c $\dfrac{75}{150}$ 1d $\dfrac{100}{250}$

1e $\dfrac{1600}{8000}$ 1f $\dfrac{120}{150}$ 1g $\dfrac{1250}{1600}$ 1h $\dfrac{18}{3}$

Answers to all the activities are at the end of the chapter (page 178).

To simplify a larger number, for example $\dfrac{800}{1600}$

it is easier to divide the top and bottom figures by 100 (i.e. delete the zeros) leaving

$$\frac{8}{16} \quad = \quad \frac{1}{2}$$

Changing fractions to decimals

To change a fraction into a decimal, divide the top number by the bottom number. For example,

$$\frac{1}{4} \quad \text{becomes} \quad 4\overline{\smash{)}1.00} = 0.25$$

Activity

Change the following to decimals:

2a $\dfrac{1}{5}$ 2b $\dfrac{1}{2}$ 2c $\dfrac{1}{10}$

Decimals

Drugs are usually administered in:

- grams (g);
- milligrams (mg);

- micrograms (µg);
- millilitres (ml).

1 kilogram (kg)	=	1000 grams
1 gram (g)	=	1000 milligrams
1 milligram (mg)	=	1000 micrograms
1 litre (l)	=	1000 millilitres

To carry out drug calculations it may be necessary to convert one unit to another. For example, if the strength of the dose you have is in milligrams, the end calculation must also be in milligrams. Thus, you would first have to convert the dose required to milligrams. *Remember* these units are SI units and therefore always increase or decease in multiples of 1000.

Multiplication of decimals

Multiplication by 10, 100, 1000, etc. can be done by simply moving the decimal point:

To multiply by	Move the decimal point
10	1 place to the right
100	2 places to the right
1000	3 places to the right

For example:

2.0 x 1000 = 2000   Decimal point moved 3 places to the right.

1.3 x 100 = 130   Decimal point moved 2 places to the right.

0.6 x 10 = 6   Decimal point moved 1 place to the right.

Activity

Try the following:

3a 0.075 × 10	**3b** 0.003 × 100	**3c** 0.01 × 1000
3d 0.2 × 1000	**3e** 0.0505 × 100	**3f** 7.7 × 1000

Division of decimals

To divide decimals by 10, 100, 1000, etc., move the point the other way – to the left.

To divide by	Move the decimal point
10	1 place to the left
100	2 places to the left
1000	3 places to the left

For example:

$37.8 \div 10 = 3.78$ Decimal point moved 1 place to the left.

$37.8 \div 100 = 0.378$ Decimal point moved 2 places to the left.

$37.8 \div 1000 = 0.0378$ Decimal point moved 3 places to the left.

Drug calculation formula

The formula to calculate a dose of medication to be administered is:

$$\frac{\text{what you want}}{\text{what you've got}} \times \frac{\text{what it's in}}{1}$$

For example; if you have 80 mg in 10 ml and you want 200 mg:

$$\frac{200}{80} \times \frac{10}{1} = 25 \text{ ml}$$

As previously stated it is essential that the units are the same throughout the calculation. For example, if you have 4 g in 250 ml and you require 800 mg, you need to convert the 4 g to milligrams first before applying the formula:

then 4 g = 4000 mg

$$\frac{800}{4000} \times \frac{250}{1} = \quad 50 \text{ ml}$$

Activity

Complete these drug calculations:

Dose ordered	Stock amp/soln
4a Ampicillin 350 mg	500 mg in 100 ml
4b Pethidine 125 mg	100 mg in 1 ml
4c Phenobarbitone 140 mg	200 mg in 1 ml
4d Heparin 1250 units	25,000 units in 1 ml
4e Potassium Chloride 16 mmol	26 mmol in 10 ml
4f Digoxin 150 μg	55 μg in 2 ml
4g Scopolamine 0.3 mg	0.4 mg in 1 ml
4h Methicillin 1750 mg	1 g in 2.5 ml

Timing the infusion

Intravenous fluids should be prescribed in millilitres but, if they are prescribed in litres, this must be converted to millilitres before any calculation is performed. British Standard adult infusion sets give 15, 20 or 60 drops per ml.

Blood sets	=	15 drops per ml (when blood is transfused)
Solutions sets	=	20 drops per ml
Burette sets	=	60 drops per ml

The formula to calculate the drops per minute is:

$$\frac{\text{volume of fluid to be infused (in ml)}}{\text{number of hours}} \times \frac{\text{number of drops per ml of giving set}}{60}$$

Round calculations down to the nearest whole number. For example, if 500 ml of Normal Saline is to be infused over 4 hours using a 20 drops per ml set, the rate is:

$$\frac{500}{4} \times \frac{20}{60} = 41 \text{ drops per minute}$$

Activity

Complete the following calculations.

- For a standard 20 drops per ml infusion set, calculate the number of drops per minute to infuse the following:

  5a 300 ml over 4 hours　　　　**5b** 145 ml over 1 hour

  5c 500 ml over 2.5 hours　　　 **5d** 800 ml over 6 hours

  5e 300 ml over 3 hours

- For a blood administration set (15 drops per ml), calculate the following in drops per minute:

  6a 150 ml over 2 hours　　　　**6b** 375 ml over 6 hours

  6c 225 ml over 3 hours　　　　**6d** 125 ml over 2 hours

  6e 165 ml over 2.5 hours

- For a paediatric burette set (60 drops per ml), calculate the drip rates to infuse the following:

  7a 320 ml over 4 hours　　　　**7b** 125 ml over 1 hour

  7c 250 ml over 4 hours　　　　**7d** 150 ml over 1 hour

  7e 50 ml over 30 minutes

DRUG ABBREVIATIONS

Abbreviation	Latin	Meaning
ac	ante cibum	before meals
ad lib	ad libitum	freely
alte die		alternate days
am	ante meridiem	morning
bid/bd	bis in die /bisdie	twice a day
c	cum	with
cap		capsule
ext		external use
gtt		drops
m	mitte	send
mg		milligrams
ml		millilitres
nocte		at night
od	omni die	once a day
o		oral/by mouth
pc	post cibum	after meals
pm	post meridiem	evening
po		by mouth/oral
prn	pro re nata	as needed/required
qds	quater in die	four times a day
s	sine	without
stat	statim	at once/straight away
tab		tablet
tds	ter die sumendum	three times a day
top		apply topically to body
ut dict	ut dictum	as directed

Useful websites

- www.nmc-uk.org
- www.bnf.org
- www.resus.org.uk
- www.mhra.gov.uk
- www.rpsgb.org.uk
- http://emc.medicines.org.uk
- www.bbc.co.uk/crime/drugs/drugsandthelaw.shtml
- www.npsa.nhs.uk
- www.cks.library.nhs.uk/clinical_knowledge/cks-drugs

Drug calculation answers

1a $\dfrac{3}{7}$	**1b** $\dfrac{2}{3}$	**1c** $\dfrac{1}{2}$	**1d** $\dfrac{2}{5}$
1e $\dfrac{1}{5}$	**1f** $\dfrac{4}{5}$	**1g** $\dfrac{25}{32}$	**1h** 6

2a 0.2 **2b** 0.5 **2c** 0.1

3a 0.75 **3b** 0.3 **3c** 10 **3d** 200

3e 5.05 **3f** 7700

4a 70 ml **4b** 1.25 ml **4c** 0.7 ml **4d** 0.05 ml

4e 6.15 ml **4f** 5.45 ml **4g** 0.75 ml **4h** 4.38 ml

Infusion rate answers

5a 25 **5b** 48.3 **5c** 66.6 **5d** 44.4

5e 33.3

6a 18.75 **6b** 15.6 **6c** 18.75 **6d** 15.6

6e 16.5

7a 80 **7b** 125 **7c** 62.5 **7d** 150

7e 100

Appendix

PRINCIPLES AND CONTENT OF AN OVERSEAS NURSING PROGRAMME (NMC, 2005c)

Principles for the programme

The development of overseas nursing programmes is based on five principles:

1 Ensure safe and effective practice in the interest of public protection.
2 Enable applicants who meet initial requirements to transfer skills and experience to the UK setting.
3 Enable applicants to be assessed as being at least as competent as any newly registered UK-trained nurse.
4 Enable supervised practice to be delivered over variable timeframes, as determined by the NMC, and based on an applicant's training and experience. The programme must also ensure that applicants meet the practice requirements for registration.
5 Be subject to NMC quality assurance processes.

Content for the programme

Content for the programme will include:

- the UK as a multicultural society;
- structure of the NHS and social care services;
- relationship between the NHS and the independent sector;
- changing health care environment;
- practitioner – client relationships;
- patient involvement in the NHS and independent sectors;
- effective communication;
- code of professional conduct;
- accountability;
- legal framework within which care is delivered;

- ethical issues;
- clinical governance and how the NMC's standards contribute to this;
- evidence-based practice;
- holistic care encompassing health promotion and education;
- multidisciplinary team working;
- numeracy skills.

References

Acheson, D (1998) *Report of the independent inquiry into inequalities in health*. London: HMSO

Aggleton, P (1990) *Health*. London: Routledge

Andrews, M and Boyle, J (1999) *Transcultural concepts in nursing care*. London: Lippincott

Auty, B (1995) 'Types of infusion pump and their risks'. *British Journal of Intensive Care*, Feb. suppl. 11–16

Baggott, R (2004) *Health and health care in Britain* (3rd edn). New York: Palgrave Macmillan

Banks, S (2004) *Ethics, accountability and the social professions*. New York: Palgrave Macmillan

Barrett, G, Sellman, D and Thomas, J (2005) *Multi-disciplinary working in health care and social care – professional perspectives*. New York: Palgrave Macmillan

Beauchamp, T and Childress, J (2001) *Principles of biomedical ethics* (5th edn). Oxford: Oxford University Press

Becker, MH (ed) (1974) *The health belief model and personal health behaviour*. New Jersey: Thorofare

Becker, MH and Maiman, LA (1975) 'Socio-behavioural determinants of compliance with medical care recommendations'. *Medical Care, xiii:* 10–24

Benner, P (1984) *From novice to expert*. California: Addison-Wesley

Black, D, Morris, J, Smith, C and Townsend, P (1980) *Inequalities in health: report of a research working group*. London: Department of Health and Social Security

Boud, D, Keogh, R and Walkwe, D (1985) *Reflection: turning experience into learning*. London: Kogan Page

Brown, R (1995) *Portfolio development and profiling for nurses*. London: Quay Books

Burnard, P and Chapman, C (2003) *Professional and ethical issues in nursing* (3rd edn). London: Balliere Tindall

Burnard, P and Kendrick, K (1998) *Ethical counselling: a workbook for nurses*. London: Edward Arnold

Campbell, H, Hothkiss, R, Bradshaw, N and Poteous, M (1998) 'Integrated Care Pathways'. *British Medical Journal*, 316: 133–137

Castledine, G (1991) 'Accountability in delivering care'. *Nursing Standard*, 5: 28–30

Caulfield, H (2005) *Vital notes for nurses: accountability*. Oxford: Blackwell

Cheung, P (1986) 'Learning your tables'. *Nursing Times*, 82: 40–41

Clark, J and Copcutt, L (1997) *Management for nurses and health care professionals.* Edinburgh: Churchill Livingstone

Clarke, P (1991) 'Towards a conceptual framework for developing interdisciplinary teams in gerentology: cognitive and ethical'. *Gerentology and Geriatrics Education,* 12: 79–96

Clarke, PB (1993) *The world's religions.* London: Readers Digest

Colyer, H and Kamath, P (1999) 'Evidence-based practice. A philosophical and political analysis: some matters for consideration by professional practitioners'. *Journal of Advanced Nursing*, 29: 188–193, in Palfreyman, S, Tod, S and Doyle, J (2003) 'An integrated approach to Evidence Based Practice'. *The Foundation of Nursing Studies Dissemination Series*, 1: 1–4

Cooper, M (1995) 'Can a zero defects philosophy be applied to drug errors?' *Journal of Advanced Nursing,* 21: 487–491

Cowley, S (ed) (2002) *Public health in policy and practice: a sourcebook for health visitors and community nurses.* London: Balliere Tindall

Craig, J and Smyth, R (2003) *The Evidence-Based Practice manual.* Edinburgh: Churchill Livingstone

Department for Constitutional Affairs (2006) *A guide to the Human Rights Act 1998: Third Edition.* London: DCA

Department of Health (1989) *Working for patients.* London: HMSO

Department of Health (1991) *The patients charter.* London: HMSO

Department of Health (1993) *A vision for the future: the nursing, midwifery and health visiting contribution to health and health care.* London: HMSO

Department of Health (1995) *Research and development: towards an evidence based health service.* London: HMSO

Department of Health (1997) *The new NHS: modern and dependable.* London: HMSO

Department of Health (1998a) A *first class service – improving quality in the new NHS.* London: Department of Health

Department of Health (1998b) *Reducing health inequalities: an action report.* London: HMSO

Department of Health (1999a) *Caldicott guardians.* London: Department of Health

Department of Health (1999b) *Making a difference.* London: Department of Health

Department of Health (1999c) *Saving lives: our healthier nation.* London: HMSO

Department of Health (1999d) *Review of prescribing, supply and administration of medicines: final report.* London: Department of Health

Department of Health (2000a) *The NHS plan: a plan for investment; a plan for reform.* London: Department of Health

Department of Health (2000b) *An organization with a memory: report of an expert group on learning from adverse events in the NHS.* London: Department of Health

Department of Health (2000c) *No secrets: guidance on developing and implementing multi-agency policies and procedures to protect vulnerable adults from abuse.* London: Department of Health

Department of Health (2000d) *The Care Standards Act.* London: HMSO

Department of Health (2001a) *Reference guide to consent for examination or treatment*. London: Department of Health

Department of Health (2001b) *Building a safer NHS for patients: implementing an organization with a memory*. London: Department of Health

Department of Health (2001c) *The essence of care; patient focused benchmarking for health care practitioners*. London: Department of Health

Department of Health (2001d) *The Health and Social Care Act*. London: Department of Health

Department of Health (2003a) *Essence of care: patient focused benchmarks for clinical governance*. London: NHS Modernisation Agency

Department of Health (2003b) *Modern matrons – improving the patient experience*. London: HMSO

Department of Health (2004a) *Choosing health: making healthy choices easier*. London: HMSO

Department of Health (2004b) *Building a safer NHS for patients: improving medication safety*. London: Department of Health

Department of Health (2005) *National strategic partnership forum – statement of purpose*. London: Department of Health

Department of Health (2006a) *Health reform in England: update and commissioning framework*. London: Department of Health

Department of Health (2006b) *Essence of care: benchmarks for promoting health*. London: Department of Health

Dimond, B (2005) *Legal aspects of nursing* (4th edn). London: Pearson Longman

Dougherty, L and Lamb, J (1999) *Intravenous therapy in nursing practice*. Edinburgh: Churchill Livingstone

Dowding, L and Barr, J (2002) *Managing in health care*. Harlow: Pearson Education

Downie, RS, Tannahill, C and Tannahill A (1998) *Health promotion – models and values*. Oxford: Oxford University Press

Driscoll, J (1994) 'Reflective practice for practice'. *Senior Nurse*, 14: 47–50

Driscoll, J (2000) *Practicing clinical supervision*. London: Balliere Tindall

ENB/Department of Health (2001) *Preparation of mentors and teachers – a new framework guidance*. London: ENB/Department of Health

ETR Associates (2005) Available from **www.etr.org/recapp/theories** (accessed 27/2/06)

European Resuscitation Council (2005) Available from **www.resus.org.uk** (accessed January 07)

Ewles, L and Simnett, I (1992) *Promoting health a practical guide* (2nd edn). London: Scutari Press

Ewles, L and Simnett, I (1999) *Promoting health a practical guide* (4th edn). London: Balliere Tindall

Fitzgerald, M (2000) 'Clinical supervision and reflective practice', in Bulman, C and Burns, S (eds) *Reflective practice in nursing* (2nd edn), ch 5. Oxford: Blackwell Scientific

Freeth, D (2001) Sustaining interprofesional collaboration. *Journal of Multi-disciplinary Care*, 15: 37–46

Funnell, P (1995) 'Exploring the value of interprofessional shared learning', in Soothill, K, Mackay, L and Webb, C *Interprofessional Relations in Health Care*, 163–171. London: Edward Arnold

Geiger, J and Davidhizar, R (1995) *Transcultural nursing: assessment and intervention.* New York: Mosby

Gerrish, K and Lacey, A (2006) *The research process in nursing.* Oxford: Blackwell

Gibbs, G (1988) *Learning by doing: a guide to teaching and learning methods.* Oxford: Further Education Unit, Oxford Polytechnic

Giddens, A (1989) *Sociology.* Oxford: Polity Press

Gillon, R (1985) *Philosophical medical ethics.* Chichester: Wiley

Gott, M and O'Brien, M (1990) 'Attitudes and belief in health promotion'. *Nursing Standard*, 5: 30–32

Health Care Commission (2005) *About the Health Care Commission* (2nd edn) London: HCC

Henley, A and Schott, J (1999) *Culture, religion and patient care in a multi-ethnic society. A handbook for professionals.* London: Age Concern

Henneman, E, Lee, J and Cohen, J (1995) 'A concept analysis of collaboration'. *Journal of Advanced Nursing*, 21: 103–109

Hofstede, G (1991) *Cultures and organisations: software of the mind.* New York: McGraw Hill

Hornby, S and Atkins, J (2000) *Collaborative care: multi-disciplinary, interagency and interpersonal* (2nd edn). Oxford: Blackwell Science

HSC (1999) *Continuing professional development (quality in the new NHS).* London: Department of Health (1999/194)

Illich, I (1977) *Limits to medicine.* London: Pelican

Independent Schools Council (2007) 'Adapting to British Culture'. **www.isc.co.uk/Internationalzone-AdaptingtoBritishCulture**

Irwin, P and Fordham, J (1995) *Evaluating the quality of care.* Edinburgh: Churchill Livingstone

Irwin, R (2007) 'Culture shock: negotiating feelings in the field'. *Anthropology Matters Journal*, 9(1) pp. 1–11

Jasper, M (2003) *Beginning reflective practice – foundations in nursing and health care.* Cheltenham: Nelson Thornes

Johns, C. 2002. *Guided reflection: advancing practice.* Oxford: Blackwell

Jones, L (1994) *The social context of health and health work.* Basingstoke: Macmillan

Laing and Buisson (2001) *Laing's healthcare market review* 2001/2002. London: Laing and Buisson

Leathard, A (1994) *Going multi-disciplinary: working together for health and welfare.* London: Routledge

Leathard, A (2003) *Interprofessional collaboration: from policy to practice in health and social care.* Hove: Brunner-Routledge

Leininger, M and McFarland, M (2002) *Transcultural nursing* (3rd edn). New York: McGraw Hill

London School of Economics and Political Science (2000) 'The Beveridge Report and the welfare state' **www.lsc.ac.ukresources/LSEHistory/beveridge_report.htm**

McClarey, M and Duff, L (1997) 'Clinical effectiveness and evidence-based practice'. *Nursing Standard*, 11: 31–35

Macqueen, CE, Brynes, AE and Frost, GS (1999) 'Treating obesity: can the stages of change model help predict outcome measures'. *Journal of Human Nutrition and Dietetics*, 12: 229–236

Mallett, J and Dougherty, L (eds) (2000) *Manual of clinical nursing procedures, Royal Marsden Hospital.* Oxford: Blackwell

Marr, H and Giebing, H (1994) *Quality assurance in nursing: concepts, methods and case studies.* Oxford: Campion Press

Middleton, S, Barnett, J and Reeves, D (2003) *What is an integrated care pathway?* Hayward Medical Communications, available from **www.evidence-based-medicine.co.uk** (accessed 12/4/07)

Miller, C, Freeman, M and Ross, N (2001) *Interprofessional practice in health and social care: challenging the shared learning agenda.* London: Edward Arnold

Milligan, F (2003) 'Adverse health-care events: Part 1. The nature of the problem'. *Professional Nurse*, 18: 502–505

Molyneux, J (2001) 'Multi-disciplinary teamworking: what makes teams work well?' *Journal of Multi-disciplinary Care*, 15: 29–35

Naidoo, J and Wills, J (2000) *Health promotion foundations for practice* (2nd edn). London: Balliere Tindall

National Council for Palliative Care (2005) *Guidance to the Mental Capacity Act 2005.* **www.ncpc.org.uk** (accessed 14 April 2007)

National Institute for Health and Clinical Excellence (NICE) (2007a) **www.nice.org.uk** (accessed 23/3/07)

National Institute for Health and Clinical Excellence (NICE) (2007b) **www.nice.org.uk/pdf/BestPracticeClinicalAudit.pdf** (accessed 21/3/07)

NHS Executive (1993) *Clinical supervision – a resource pack.* London: Department of Health

NHS Executive (1994) *The evolution of clinical audit.* London: HMSO

Nursing and Midwifery Admissions Service (NMAS) (2007) Available from **www.nmas.ac.uk/apply.html** (accessed April 2007)

Nursing and Midwifery Council (2001) *Clinical supervision.* London: NMC

Nursing and Midwifery Council (2004a) *Code of professional conduct: standards for conduct, performance and ethics.* London: NMC

Nursing and Midwifery Council (2004b) *Guidelines for the administration of medicines.* London: NMC

Nursing and Midwifery Council (2004c) *Standards of proficiency for pre-registration nursing education.* London: NMC

Nursing and Midwifery Council (2005a) *Guidelines for records and record-keeping.* London: NMC

Nursing and Midwifery Council (2005b) *Changing policy, changing practice.* London: NMC

Nursing and Midwifery Council (2005c) *Supporting nurses and midwives through lifelong learning.* London: NMC

Nursing and Midwifery Council (2005d) *Requirements for overseas nurses' programme leading to registration in the UK, Circular 9-2005 Appendix 1*. London: NMC

Nursing and Midwifery Council (2006a) *The PREP Handbook*. London: NMC

Nursing and Midwifery Council (2006b) *Clinical governance advice sheet*. Available from **www.nmc-org.uk** (accessed 17/5/07)

Nursing and Midwifery Council (2006c) *Standards to support learning and assessment in practice*. London: NMC

Nursing and Midwifery Council (2006d) *Preceptorship*. London: NMC

Nursing and Midwifery Council (2007a) *Registrant/client relationships and the prevention of abuse*. Available from **www.nmc-org.uk** (accessed 16/5/07)

Nursing and Midwifery Council (2007b) *Medicines management (A–Z advice sheet)*. Available from **www.nmc-org.uk** (accessed May 2007)

Office for National Statistics (2007) *National statistics on line*. Available from **www.statistics.gov.uk** (accessed 12/5/07)

Office of Population Censuses and Surveys (2001) Available from **www.gov.uk** (accessed 21/2/06).

Offredy, M (2006) 'Evidence based practice', in Peate, I *Becoming a nurse in the 21st century*. Chichester: Wiley

O'Rourke, A (2005) 'Minimising clinical risk', *Current Paediatrics*, 15: 466–472

Palfreyman, S, Tod, S and Doyle, J (2003) 'An integrated approach to Evidence Based Practice'. *The Foundation of Nursing Studies Dissemination Series*, 1: 1–4

Papadopoulos, I, Tilki, M and Taylor, G (1998) *Transcultural care: a guide for health care professionals*. London: Quay Books

Parahoo, K (2006) *Nursing research principles, process and issues*. New York: Palgrave Macmillan

Pearsall, J (ed) (2001) *The concise Oxford dictionary* (10th edn revised). Oxford: Oxford University Press

Peate, I (2006) *Becoming a nurse in the 21st century*. Chichester: Wiley

Pietroni, P (1992) 'Towards reflective practice – the languages of health and social care'. *Journal of Interprofessional Care*, 1: 7–16

Price, B (2002) 'Effective learning no. 3: reflective observations in practice'. *Nursing Standard*, 17: S1–2

Prochaska, J and DiClemente, C (1984) *The transtheoretical approach: crossing traditional foundations of change*. Harnewood: Don Jones/Irwin

Richards, A and Edwards, S (2003) *A nurses survival guide to the ward*. Edinburgh: Churchill Livingstone

Roden, J (2004) 'Revisiting the Health Belief Model: nurses applying it to young families and their health promotion needs'. *Nursing and Health Sciences*, 6: 1–10

Rosenstock, I (1966) 'Why people use health services'. *Milbank Memorial Fund Quarterly*, 44: 94–121

Royal College of General Practitioners (2004) *The structure of the NHS. Information sheet no 8*. London: RCGP

Royal College of Nursing (1996) *The Royal College of Nursing clinical effectiveness initiative – A strategic framework*. London: RCN

Royal College of Nursing (2002) *Clinical supervision in the workplace: guidance for occupational health nurses*. London: RCN

Royal College of Nursing (2003) *Clinical governance: an RCN resource guide*. London: RCN

Royal College of Nursing (2004) *The future nurse: the future for nurse education*. London: RCN

Royal College of Nursing (2005) *Methicillin-resistant Staphylococcus aureus (MRSA): guidance for nursing staff*. London: RCN

Royal College of Nursing (2006) *Transcultural health care practice: an educational resource for nurses and health care practitioners*. Available from **www.rcn.org.uk/resources/transcultural/index.php** (accessed 21/2/06)

Sackett, D, Richardson, S and Rosenberg, W (1997) *Evidence-based medicine: how to practice and teach*. Edinburgh: Churchill Livingstone

Sackett, D, Richardson, S, Rosenberg, W and Haynes, R (2000) *Evidence-based medicine. How to teach and practice* (2nd edn). Edinburgh: Churchill Livingstone

Sackett, D, Rosenberg, W, Muir Gray, J and Richardson, S (1996) 'Evidence-based medicine: What it is and what it isn't'. *British Journal of Medicine*, 312: 71–72

Sale, D (2000) *Quality assurance: a pathway to excellence*. Basingstoke: Macmillan

Sale, D (2005) *Understanding clinical governance and quality assurance*. New York: Palgrave Macmillan

Scottish Executive (2000) *Our national health: a plan for action, a plan for change*. Edinburgh: Scottish Executive

Scriven, A and Orme, J (2001) *Health promotion professional perspectives* (2nd edn). New York: Palgrave Macmillan

Seedhouse, D (1986) *Health: the foundations for achievement*. Chichester: Wiley

Seedhouse, D (1997) *Health promotion: philosophy, prejudice and practice*. Chichester: Wiley

Shannon, C, Weaver, W (1949) *A Mathematical Theory of Communication*. Illinois: University of Illinois Press.

Sharp, A and Howard, K (1996) *The management of a student research project* (2nd edn). Aldershot: Gower

Solomon, J (2003) 'Eating and drinking', in Holland, K, Jenkins, J, Solomon, J and Whittam, S (eds) (2003) *Roper, Logan and Tierny Model in practice*. Edinburgh: Churchill Livingstone

Somerset Academy (2005) *Reflective framework*. Taunton: Somerset Academy

Soothill, K, Mackay, L and Webb, C (1995) *Multi-disciplinary relations in health care*. London: Edward Arnold

Stapleton, SR (1998) 'Team-building: making collaborative practice work'. *Journal of Midwifery*, 43: 12–18.

Stead, CK (ed) (1977) *The letters and journals of Katherine Mansfield: a selection*. London: Allen Lane

Stephenson, S (1994) 'Reflection – a student perspective', in Palmer, A, Burns, S and Bulman, C (eds) *Reflective practice in nursing: the growth of the professional practitioner*. Oxford: Blackwell

Tingle, J and Cribb, A (2006) *Nursing law and ethics*. Oxford: Blackwell

Torn, A and McNichol, E (1998) 'A qualitative study utilizing a focus group to explore the role and concept of the nurse practitioner'. *Journal of Advanced Nursing*, 27: 1202–1211.

Tschudin, V (2003) *Ethics in nursing: the caring relationship*. London: Butterworth Heinemann

UKCC (1996) *Position statement on clinical supervision for nursing and health visiting*. London: UKCC

UKCC (1999) *Fitness for practice*. London: UKCC

UKCC (2002) *Report on higher level of practice project*. London: UKCC

Wagner, AL (2002) 'Nursing students' development of caring through creative reflective practice', in Freshwater, D (ed) *Theraputic nursing: improving patient care through self awareness and reflection*. London: Sage

Waitt, C, Waitt, P and Pirmohame, DM (2004) 'Intravenous therapy'. *Postgraduate Medical Journal*, 80: 1–6

Weller, P (ed) (1997) *Religions in the UK: a multi-faith directory*. Derby: University of Derby

Welsh Assembly Government (2001) *Improving health in Wales*. Cardiff: National Assembly

Whitehead, D (2000) 'The role of the community based nurse in health promotion'. *British Journal of Community Nursing*, 5: 604–608

Whitehead, E and Mason, T (2003) *Study skills for nurses*. London: Sage

Wikipedia (2006) *Communication*. Available from **www.En.wikipedia.org/wiki/Communication** (accessed 9/3/06)

Wilson-Barnett, J, Macleo, and Clarke, K (eds) (1993) *Research in health promotion and Nursing*. Basingstoke: Macmillan

World Health Organisation (1986) *Ottawa charter for health promotion: an international conference on health promotion*, November 17–21. Copenhagen: WHO

Wright, K (2005) 'An exploration into the most effective way to teach drug calculation skills to nursing students'. *Nurse Education Today*, 25: 430–436

Websites references

National Institute for Health and Clinical Excellence
www.nice.org.uk/page.aspx?o=guidance (accessed 23/3/07)

NHS Direct
www.nhsdirect.nhs.uk (accessed 23/3/07)

London School of Economics and Political Science (2000) 'The Beveridge Report and the welfare state'
www.lse.ac.uk/resorces/LSEHistory?beveridge_report (accessed 25/4/07)

Department of Health
www.dh.gov.uk/en/policyandguidance (accessed 24/3/07)

National Statistics
www.statistics.gov.uk (accessed 17/5/07)

UK Data Archive
www.data-archive.ac.uk (accessed 17/5/07)

Wikipedia
ww.wikipedia.org (accessed 17/5/07)

Independent Schools Council
www.isc.co.uk/InternationalZone_AdaptingtoBritishCulture (accessed 17/5/07)

Ethnicity Online
www.ethnicityonline.net/ethnic_groups,htm (accessed 17/5/07)

UK Council for International Student Affairs
www.ukcosa.org.uk/images/shock (accessed 20/8/07

Arizona State University
www.asu.edu/clas/shesc/projects/bajaethnography/shock (accessed 20/8/07)

Commission for Patient and Public Involvement in Health
www.cppih.org/about_what.html (accessed 23/3/2007)

Citizens Advice Bureau
www.adviceguide.org.uk/index/family_parent/health/nhs_complaints.htm (accessed 23/3/07)

National Patient Safety Agency
www.npsa.nhs.uk (accessed 23/3/07)

Commission for Social Care Inspection
www.csci.org.uk/about_csci.aspx (accessed 23/03/07)

Patient Advice and Liaison Service
www.pals.nhs.uk/splash.ASPX?NodeId=4 (accessed 27/3/07)

The Patients' Forum
www.thepatientsforum.org.uk/aboutpf.asp (accessed 27/3/07)

Chartered Society of Physiotherapy
www.csp.org.uk (accessed 12/4/07)

Department of Health
www.dh.gov.uk (accessed 5/1/07)

International Council of Nurses
www.icn.ch/definition.htm (accessed 5/1/07)

Nursing and Midwifery Council
www.nmc-uk.org (accessed 5/1/07)

National Health Service Clinical Knowledge Summaries
www.prodigy.nhs.uk (accessed 5/1/07)

Skills for Health
www.skillsforhealth.org.uk/careerframework/key_elements.php

National Health Service Modernisation Agency
www.wise.nhs.uk (accessed 5/1/07)

National Health Service Careers
www.nhscareers.nhs.uk/nhs-knowledge_base/ data/7806.html (accessed 18/4/07)

National Health Service Careers
www.nhscareers.nhs.uk/nhs-knowledge_base/ data/5632.html (accessed 18/4/07)

Learn Direct
www.learndirect-advice.co.uk/helpwithyourcareer/jobprofiles/profiles/profile709
(accessed 18/4/07)

General Social Care Council
www.gscc.org.uk/Training+and+learning/Become+a+social+worker/Becoming+a+
social+worker+FAQs (accessed 18/4/07)

Prospects Graduate Careers
www.prospects.ac.uk/cms/ShowPage/Home_page/Explore_types_of_jobs/Type
(accessed 18/4/07)

American Academy of Family Physicians
www.aafp.org/afp/200000301/1409html (accessed 3/4/07)

EngenderHealth
www.engenderhealth.org/res/onc/sti/preventings/sti6p2.html (accessed 3/4/07)

Index